The Emmanuel Movement
Boston, 1904–1929

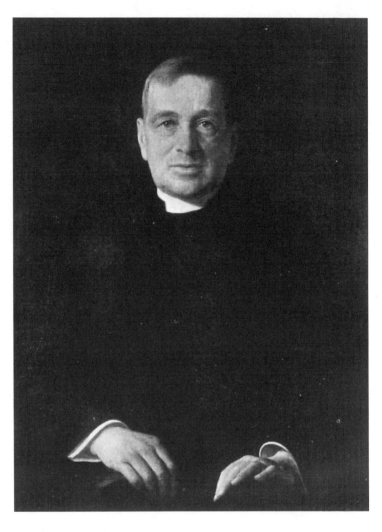

Oil portrait of the Reverend Elwood Worcester, painted by Emil Pollak-Ottendorf in 1917. Reproduced from the frontispiece in his autobiography, *Life's Adventure*, 1932.

The Emmanuel Movement

(Boston, 1904–1929)

The Origins of Group Treatment
and
The Assault on Lay
Psychotherapy

Sanford Gifford

Distributed by the Harvard University Press for
The Francis Countway Library of Medicine, Boston, 1997

ISBN: 0-674-25111-3

Contents

Illustrations

Robert Thaxter Edes and Frederick Henry Gerrish

Photographs of Joseph H. Pratt's "fresh air treatment" of tuberculosis

Joseph H. Pratt examining patients at his tuberculosis clinic, ca. 1912

Constance Worcester; Dr. Blandina Worcester; Entrance of the former Emmanuel Church rectory

Preface

This monograph on the Rev. Elwood Worcester and the Emmanuel Movement evolved from the author's brief biographical sketch of Dr. Isador Coriat, an early collaborator of Dr. Worcester's in the Emmanuel Movement, and later president of the second Boston Psychoanalytic Society. I wrote this sketch in 1969, primarily because members of our Society knew so little about our founding fathers, including Coriat. Further readings in Coriat's lively scrapbooks, which included three volumes of a national clipping service for the years 1906–53, prompted me to write a short version of this present study in 1970. A longer version was written a year later, in preparation for the 1973 symposium, "Psychoanalysis, Psychotherapy and the Boston Medical Scene, 1894–1944." An abridgment of that paper appeared in the published proceedings of the symposium.[1]

In reading Coriat's scrapbooks, my interest had been captured by vivid journalistic accounts of public controversies about the Emmanuel Movement, the new psychotherapies of suggestion, psychoanalysis, and the treatment of mental patients by non-physicians. I was also encouraged by Mr. Richard J. Wolfe, Curator of Rare Books and Manuscripts in The Countway Library, who introduced me to Dr. Russell George Vasile and lent me Vasile's honors thesis on James Jackson Putnam, Boston's first psychoanalyst, which was eventually published in 1977.[2] The year that I was exploring early analytic history, 1971, proved to be the year in which Nathan Hale published two important books: the first about James Jackson Putnam and his correspondence with Freud and Ernest Jones and the second his monumental study, *Freud in America.*[3] This was the first volume of his projected history of psychoanalysis in the United States, of which its sequel has just appeared in print.

In the intervening years I have built on these and other contributions which have appeared in print during this time to complete a clearer picture of this novel attempt to combine religion and medicine, lay psychotherapy, and early group treatment methods, and to trace the influences and parallels in later attempts to treat alcoholism and the common neuroses. I am grateful to many of these fellow-workers for their help on this study, but I will mention only a few, beginning with Dr. Marian Putnam herself, who had been a neighbor of the Worcesters on Marlborough Street in 1905. She later became a psychoanalyst, like her father, and a leading child-analyst.

Next, I would like to acknowledge the great help of the Rev. Worcester's daughters, Dr. Blandina Worcester (Mrs. Carroll Brewster), and Miss Constance Worcester, who created a half-way house for mental patients that continued her father's work until her death in 1986. In the course of my researches, Constance Worcester and I became good friends, and I served as a psychiatric consultant to some of her difficult, long-term patients.

I am also grateful for the help of Dr. Worcester's son, the late Gurdon Worcester, and to his grand-nephew, Mr. Carroll Brewster, formerly president of Hobart and William Smith College. Mr. Brewster lent me another amazing set of scrapbooks containing newspaper clippings about the Emmanuel Movement, from 1906 to 1916, which he subsequently donated to the Rare Book Collection in the Countway Medical Library. Besides the scholarly help of Mr. Wolfe and Dr. Vasile, I would also like to thank Prof. Nathan Hale, Dr. Eugene Taylor, Dr. Robert Powell and Mr. Ian Evison for helpful suggestions and out-of-the-way references over a number of years. For help in tracing the elusive history of Dr. Worcester's successor, Courtenay Baylor, I would like to acknowledge the help of Mrs. Emmeline Dunne, Ms. Nora Murphy of the Episcopal Diocesan Library in Boston, Mr. Peter Carrini of the Simmons College archives, and Prof. William Koelsch of Clark University, Worcester. Finally I am grateful to Dr. Arthur S. Pier, Constance Worcester's personal physician, for his thoughtful recollections of her life over many years, and his account of her last illness and death.

Sanford Gifford M. D.
11 November 1994.

1

The Emmanuel Movement and the Origins of Group Psychotherapy

"The Emmanuel Movement" was the name given by the contemporary press to a combined method of group and individual psychotherapy introduced in 1906 by the Rev. Elwood Worcester, Rector of the Emmanuel Church in Boston. This form of treatment for the common neuroses was offered to the public, free of charge, open to all social classes and to individuals of any religious denomination or of no religion at all. The group meetings were conducted in a basement auditorium of the church by two clergymen, Dr. Worcester himself and the Rev. Samuel McComb, with the medical supervision of an internist, Dr. Richard C. Cabot, and a psychiatrist, Dr. Isador Coriat. Worcester was unusual as a minister in that he was also a clinical psychologist. He had earned the Ph.D. degree at the University of Leipzig, studying psychology under Wilhelm Wundt and Gustav Fechner, and the Rev. McComb had had a similar graduate education in England. Worcester and

McComb's methods of individual treatment were no different from other psychotherapies of suggestion, then reaching their peak of popularity, based on hypnosis and a dynamic concept of the unconscious. Worcester's innovation was the use of weekly group-meetings, in addition to individual therapy. His group-methods had evolved from his collaboration with Dr. Joseph Pratt, an internist who had applied the "class method" to the home treatment of tuberculosis in 1905.

The Emmanuel Movement was first welcomed with great popular acclaim, because of its dramatic cures of hysterical symptoms, but its very success, and its popularity, seemed to evoke fierce public controversies. Both its initial acceptance and its subsequent decline were associated with and intensified by the kind of widespread newspaper publicity characteristic of the "new journalism." Worcester was attacked by traditional clergymen for practicing "faith healing," by Christian Scientists for collaborating with doctors, and by the medical establishment for practicing lay-psychotherapy, or the treatment of patients by non-physicians. Worcester and McComb were not physicians, but both held Ph.D. degrees in psychology, like William James, Josiah Royce and others who also practiced psychotherapy at that time. Worcester, from the beginning, had emphasized his close ties with eminent physicians like Richard Cabot and Joseph Pratt. But most physicians remained implacably hostile, including Sigmund Freud who had come to America to give his Clark University lectures in 1909, and James Jackson Putnam who became Boston's first psychoanalyst.

Widespread publicity about the Emmanuel Movement seemed to wane after 1912, but Worcester continued to work unobtrusively until his retirement in 1929, with a large and devoted following. Two of his lay assistants, Ernst Jacoby and Courtenay Baylor, applied Worcester's group-methods to the treatment of alcoholism. Their use of an ex-alcoholic peer as group-leader foreshadowed Alcoholics Anonymous and other self-help drug-treatment methods that appeared many years later, although no direct link can be traced.

In looking back on the Emmanuel Movement, the present-day reader is impressed by the originality of Worcester's group-methods as a precursor of the group-psychotherapy movement. His program of offering free treatment to patients of all faiths and social classes suggests an early experiment in "community psychotherapy." But these innovations can be better understood by examining their background in the "mind-cure" movements at the turn of the century, and in the impact of psychoanalysis which overlapped and eventually superseded the psychotherapies of suggestion. In this broader context, with its complex interactions among divergent trends in science, medicine and popular culture, the Emmanuel Movement stands out as a short but significant battle over lay-psychotherapy, in the endless wars about the right of non-physicians to treat patients. This seems a peculiarly American preoccupation, perhaps, according to Nathan Hale,[1] because American medicine was slow in establishing standards of training, compared to traditional European universities and medical schools.

At that time, oddly enough, Freud and Putnam stood together on what seemed the "wrong" side of the controversy in supporting the medical establishment against lay-psychotherapy. At all other times Freud was a staunch advocate of lay-analysis, and many European analysts were not physicians. Putnam himself appointed a non-medical psychoanalyst, L. E. Emerson, to his department at the Massachusetts General Hospital. American psychoanalysis has been continuously tormented by battles over the acceptance of non-M.D.s for analytic training from its beginnings until very recently. What Freud called our "medical fixation" set American analysis apart from analysis in every other country in the world. Finally, the American Psychoanalytic Association took steps to resolve the conflict, by voting for the Gaskill Proposal[2] to accept non-physicians for full analytic training. But the final vote of the Association was not taken until 1991.

An important feature of late nineteenth century life in America was an apparently increased incidence of the neuroses, fatigue-states called neurasthenia, neurotic depressions and the somatic manifestations of hysteria, called "functional disorders." Since the 1880s George Beard[3] had explained neurasthenia as a "disease of civilization," and thus a typically American affliction, he believed, because the United States exemplified the competitive demands of modern life in their most intense form. Whether this increase in neurotic illness was real or based on greater public recognition of these disorders cannot be determined; there is no doubt, however, that the demand for treatment had greatly increased in the United States. This occurred at a time when psychiatrists were very few, and, with a few exceptions like Adolf Meyer and William A. White, they were isolated in state mental hospitals for the custodial care of the insane. Thus the treatment of the neuroses fell upon family doctors, internists, surgeons and neurologists, because so many manifestations of neurosis presented in the form of physical symptoms.

In the 1880s, the new methods of treatment were hypnosis and other forms of suggestion, first put to practical use by the French neurologists Charcot, Bernheim and Janet. Freud was among the few Europeans outside of France to study the uses of suggestion in treating neuroses, and, with the collaboration of Breuer, he evolved his own method, which came to be called psychoanalysis. The pre-analytic methods of suggestion were very appealing to Americans, and to Bostonians in particular, among neurologists like James Jackson Putnam and Morton Prince, psychologists like William James, and internists and surgeons like Robert Edes and Henry Gerrish. All shared some concept of unconscious mental activity, called the "subconscious" or the "subliminal," in contrast to Freud's concept of "the system Unconscious." The treatment-methods associated with what came to be called "the psychotherapy movement" were hypnosis, "waking suggestion" and moral re-education, borrowed from Déjerine and Dubois. These trends can be seen most clearly in Boston between 1890, when James wrote *The Hidden Self*,[4] and 1909, when Freud gave his introductory lectures at Clark University.[5]

We now recognize more clearly that Freudian analysis was first welcomed in this country as merely another form of suggestive therapy. And the great public enthusiasm for both the pre-analytic psychotherapy movement and for psychoanalysis owed something to characteristic features of American life. One was the persistent hold of religion on the popular imagination, as in the recurrent waves of evangelistic fervor that had swept the country throughout the nineteenth century. These religious movements were superseded by secularized philosophic equivalents of religion that took the form of Transcendentalism, various Utopian social movements, and the many ethical and philanthropic reform-movements of the Progressive Era.[6] Similar recurrent patterns of enthusiasm can be found in the reception of both scientific and pseudo-scientific discoveries, embraced with quasi-religious zeal and condemned with equal intensity. These episodes of public acclaim were associated with Mesmerism and Spiritualism, phrenology and homeopathy, and with many health fads like vegetarianism, Dr. Graham's crackers, and the "fresh air" cult.

There were, of course, comparable religious fervors, faith-healers and Utopian movements in Europe, but their relation to religion seemed different. In European countries with state churches, there was a traditional antagonism between science and religion, in which most scientists, from the time of Galileo, sought to establish a secular basis for their discoveries, free from moral and religious judgments. In the United States, however, with its traditional belief that each man is free to create his own religion, the same kind of person who was attracted by new religious enthusiasms was almost equally susceptible to innovations in science and political theory. Thus European scientists and social reformers tended to be agnostic or anti-clerical, and the religious to be politically conservative. While America, in contrast, generated unusual combinations of religious, scientific and political radicalism, creating some unlikely intellectual bedfellows.

Against this background, the Emmanuel Movement can be seen as an attempted synthesis between native American religious predilections and European scientific discoveries in the new psychotherapy of suggestion. After a brilliant initial success, the Emmanuel Movement foundered among the conflicting scientific cross-currents of its time, partly, in fact, because of its popularity. In the 1890s the Christian Science Church and other faith-healing sects had also gained great popularity, in response to the same increased need for the treatment of neuroses that physicians were unable to fulfill. The initial reaction of the medical profession was a defensive one, denouncing the religious elements as anti-scientific and fiercely opposing the treatment of patients by non-physicians. At the height of this controversy, the Emmanuel Movement attempted to reconcile a traditional religious setting with a new scientific method of treatment, and this evoked some unexpected and paradoxical attitudes among the cultural leaders of that era.

As I noted, Worcester was attacked by most physicians for his use of lay therapists, and yet defended by a few doctors like Cabot and Pratt, who were sympathetic to the new psychotherapies of suggestion. Putnam, a leader in the psychotherapy movement, first accepted and then attacked the Emmanuel Movement, and was soon to become Boston's first psychoanalyst. Freud also attacked the Emmanuel Movement, although he was a life-long advocate of lay-analysis. Ironically, he had just welcomed a Swiss clergyman, the Rev. Pfister, into the ranks of psychoanalysts, suggesting that Freud's well-known antipathy to religion was not the sole basis for his rejecting the Emmanuel Movement. William James had always been a defender of lay-psychotherapy, accepting physicians, psychologists and faith-healers as part of the "mind-cure" movement, and had fought the medical establishment in the Massachusetts Legislature against compulsory medical licenses for psychotherapists. He had criticized Freud for attacking the popular psychotherapy movements, and deplored the destruction of the Emmanuel Movement by its excessive newspaper publicity.

In a broader sense both the issue of lay-analysis, and the Emmanuel Movement which exemplified it, can be seen as touchstones to contemporary American public opinion. Both elicited some typical contradictory attitudes and created some unusual bedfellows, as well as adversaries. Today we are surprised to hear that Freud allied himself with conservative neurologists like E. W. Taylor against the Emmanuel Movement, while William James defended the Rev. Worcester and criticized Freud's dream theories as "a most dangerous method." And we are even more surprised when James, Worcester and Freud all shared a common interest in the current vogue for telepathy and table-rapping. But such seeming contradictions run throughout 19th century America, when Utopian socialists favored Spiritualism, Abolitionists became teetotalers and early Marxists espoused vegetarianism.

In summary, then, this study is not only a history of the Emmanuel Movement but a reexamination of its unusual position during a critical phase in the development of American psychotherapy, before and after the advent of psychoanalysis. Its origins and fate illuminate two native attitudes that differed from contemporary developments in Europe: 1) the rapid initial acceptance of psychoanalysis, which was perceived as a form of medical psychotherapy, and 2) the power of native medical orthodoxy to shape the American psychoanalytic movement, differentiating it from European tolerance for lay-analysis.

2

The Founding Father:
Elwood Worcester (1862–1940)

The founder of the Emmanuel Movement, Dr. Elwood Worcester, was born in Ohio and grew up in upper New York State, but he came from an old New England family and, at the age of forty-two, he settled permanently in Boston. He recalled his childhood in idyllic terms, living in a pastoral, pre-industrial countryside, within a loving, well-to-do family. His adolescence and student years were filled with family tragedies, Dickensian poverty and prodigious feats of hard work, that bring to mind many ingredients of nineteenth century novels and biographies.

According to Worcester's memoirs,[1] his forebears "preserved for three centuries in America some very peculiar, striking characteristics." Among them were many ministers, doctors, social reformers, and a once-famous lexicographer. The first Worcester to reach these shores arrived in 1639, an Anglican clergyman with a full set of communion silver. He soon became a Puritan pastor in Salisbury, Massachusetts. "Among wolves one must learn to howl a little," Elwood Worcester wrote about his ancestor, aptly quoting Voltaire. Toward the end of the eighteenth century, a Rev. Noah Worcester was living in Thornton, New Hampshire, where he wrote a strongly anti-Trinitarian treatise. Condemned for his heterodoxy by the Hopkinton council of Calvinist clergy, Worcester was welcomed by William Ellery Channing and invited to edit the first Unitarian journal, the *Christian Disciple.* He moved to Brighton, Massachusetts, wrote a book opposed to war in any form, and in 1815 founded the Massachusetts Peace Society.

Three of Noah Worcester's four sons became ministers, two of whom were leaders in establishing the Church of the New Jerusalem in Boston.[2] The younger son, Thomas, had discovered Swedenborg's voluminous Latin writings in the Harvard library while working his way through college by waiting on table. He formed a study group to read these works and, in 1818, he was chosen to be the first pastor of the Church of the New Jerusalem while he was still a divinity-student. For fifty-five years Thomas Worcester led, or rather dominated this heretical congregation, at first supporting the church by running a boarding-house for Swedenborgians in Louisburg Square. Later he introduced the practice of tithing its members according to their income, and advocating Swedenborg's doctrine of "conjugal love" which was misunderstood as a form of "free love." By 1848, he was warning his flock about their uncritical enthusiasm for the Utopian theories of Fourier, when a member of his congregation had proposed that a synthesis of Fourier and Swedenborg would create a perfect "union of Science and Religion," foreshadowing the Emmanuel Movement's would-be union of "Religion and Medicine."

There were many other eminent or original Worcester forbears during the nineteenth century, five of whom appeared in the *Dictionary of American Biography.*[3] Samuel

Austin Worcester was a clergyman, missionary and linguist who translated the Bible into Cherokee and set up the first Indian printing press in Oklahoma Territory. A younger Noah Worcester was a physician who studied medicine in Europe; he was said to have brought back the first stethoscope from France. The best-known Worcester was the lexicographer, Joseph Emerson Worcester, who introduced the "compromise *a*" into American speech (intermediate between *hat* and *father*). He waged and lost the "battle of the dictionaries" with Noah Webster, and was buried in Mt. Auburn Cemetery.

In Elwood Worcester's own time, his cousin Joseph was pastor of a small Swedenborgian congregation in San Francisco. Another cousin, Dr. Alfred Worcester, was a much beloved physician who was still giving fatherly talks on "sexual hygiene" to Harvard freshmen in the early 1930s. "Oddly enough," Worcester wrote about his family, "several of its physicians have also been preachers, and more than one of its ministers have also practiced medicine; so that my deep interest in the sick in mind and body came to me naturally." (This had also been true of early Puritan ministers like Cotton Mather.) He also emphasized his family's "marked tendency to mysticism" and its interest in social reform, resulting in "a family of practical mystics." Although Worcester wrote about his Swedenborgian forebears with a certain pride, he showed no interest whatever in New Church doctrine, which included both spiritualism (communication with the dead) and a belief in "Divine Healing." This is surprising, in the light of Worcester's keen interest in the Spiritualist Movement and his active participation in the Boston Society for Psychical Research.

Swedenborgianism, in fact, with its mixture of scientific and mystical elements, attracted many physicians and clergymen, as well as non-conformist intellectuals of all kinds.[4] Followers of the New Church in America were well-known for their passionate involvement in successive "causes," from Mesmerism and the emancipation of slaves at the turn of the eighteenth century, through Utopian socialism, Fourierism. spiritualism and homeopathy by 1840, to the "mind-cure" movement and New Thought in Elwood Worcester's lifetime. Despite this unconventional background, however, Worcester seemed to feel no conflict between his orthodox Episcopal training, his fashionable Back Bay parish and his innovative path in group psychotherapy.

In his memoirs, Worcester describes his grandfather as a Gloucester shipowner, who became bankrupt after two shipwrecks, and moved to Philadelphia. His father, David Freeman Worcester (1815–1880), went to work as a clerk in order to send a brilliant younger brother to college. In an engaging autobiographical sketch,[5] his father described himself at eighteen as "large and strong, and ambitious to make my way by the sweat of my brow rather than behind a counter." Moving to "what was then called 'Out West,'" a river town near Pittsburgh, he went to work for a Quaker timber-merchant. "True to his saving instincts," his employer leapt onto a raft that was being carried away by flood-waters of the Ohio, and Worcester swam after him; they landed their cargo downstream, sold it and returned with a profit.

David Worcester painted houses, taught in a female seminary and embarked on an adventurous career as trader, lumberman and land-speculator, traveling widely up and down the Ohio and Mississippi river systems. His memoirs are full of lively anecdotes about outwitting other traders, at a time when "Yankee trader" meant "wily" and "shrewd". Among his business ventures were the discovery and re-sale of coal-fields, as a self-taught geologist and prospector in Kentucky and West Virginia, and he operated canal-boats, packets and warehouses in Brooklyn. At long last he settled in Massillon, Ohio, with his wife and growing family, shortly after the crash of 1854. According to his son, he "made and lost about ten fortunes" before his death after another business failure in 1880.

Elwood Worcester was born in Massillon in 1862, when his father was forty-seven, as an only son with three older sisters. The family moved to Rochester, New York when he was two, and he recalled memories that predate that event. He was riding in a "democrat wagon" with his father, his feet resting on a fleecy white lamb, trussed up under the seat. When he asked his oldest sister what a circular clothes-line was for, she said it was a gallows for hanging naughty boys. At six he recalled the death of his favorite aunt, her body in the coffin and "the imprint of her cold, stiff lips against mine." Asking his sister what would happen after burial, he was told that his aunt would "lie in the ground forever and ever and worms would feast on her."

For years the young Worcester was preoccupied by fears of death and physical decay, and he had nightmares in which he was pursued by winged devils and floated weightlessly up and down the vast stairwell of his aunt's house. Other childhood memories included frequent teasing inflicted by this same eldest sister, who locked him in closets and helped him climb the highest trees in order to abandon him, too frightened to climb down. Once, having instructed him in lighting matches, she showed him how to set the hayloft on fire; they hid in a high willow-tree, to watch the burning barn and their parents' frantic efforts to find them until late in the evening.

He remembers his father's method of teaching him to swim at the age of six, "by throwing me into deep water and watching me struggle for the shore." Instead of a phobia, Worcester developed a great love of the water, fondly recalling reckless feats of long-distance swimming at night during college and a life-long habit of taking ice-cold baths each morning. One day on a drive, he heard his mother asking his nurse if Elwood was retarded, because he scarcely spoke by the age of three. Having understood their conversation perfectly, he amazed his mother by suddenly speaking fluently. He went on to develop an unusual verbal memory, recalling long speeches of Daniel Webster, nearly half of Goethe's *Faust,* and most of Thomson's *City of Dreadful Night,* "because something in my nature must have responded to its sombre beauty."

In spite of these grim, even traumatic memories, Worcester continued to recollect his childhood as an idyllic, blissful one. "Nothing fortifies and sustains us so much," he concluded, "as to be able to look back to noble and loving parents and to recall the unclouded heaven of our childhood happiness." He contrasted these happy memories with those of "sad, depressed, dissociated persons, the seeds of [whose] future unhappiness has been sown in childhood, not by heredity but inflicted by parents and teachers who attempt to 'break the child's will'."

Among other experiences with his father's educational methods, in addition to his regular schooling, Worcester began the study of Latin at age six and Greek at eight, at a slightly older age than John Stuart Mill submitted to his father's similar tutelage. These extra lessons were held at the dinner-table, after supper had been cleared, and included their servants, "nice jolly girls and boys who, when they came to us, could scarcely read and write." At ten he was sent to a boarding school thirty miles away, from which he walked home at Christmas one year when his parents were unable to fetch him. He learned quickly and had completed his college requirements by the age of thirteen.

At this crucial age in Elwood's life, his father suffered another bankruptcy, which Worcester called "a typical American family tragedy." His father died in 1880, when Worcester was nearly seventeen, and his mother became totally blind from glaucoma, after several unsuccessful operations. In a state of "utter prostration," she seemed unable to manage the household and took refuge in religion. Worcester recalled this family religious "awakening" as beginning with his eldest sister Mary, the one who had teased him in childhood. His memories of this period were dark and cloudy, as he and his sisters wandered about the great house and grounds, "lonely and desolate, like pygmies in the abode of giants."

As the only son, Worcester attempted to support the family, by peddling from door to door, by working as a freight-handler, and by becoming a clerk in the local railroad shipping-room. Here, one winter day, he experienced his own religious awakening, when the yellow wall of the shipping-room "suddenly seemed strangely to brighten." When this happened again, without any natural source of light, he heard a voice: "be faithful to me and I will be faithful to you." Knowing nothing at the time "of the experiences of mystics, or of the visual and auditory hallucinations collected by the Society for Psychical Research," the experience "produced an overwhelming effect on my mind, and it was destined to change my whole existence." After consulting the Rev. Algernon Crapsey, a mildly heretical local minister, Worcester embarked on a course of study. Rising each morning at five, he studied Greek composition until seven. At lunch he read passages in Grote and Mommsen, and in the Greek New Testament each evening after work.

A year or so later Worcester fell ill with typhoid fever, and after a protracted convalescence he set off for Columbia University. He had $17 and a free pass on the New York Central in his pocket, and he considered himself "more ignorant of the world than most boys of ten today." In spite of further experiences of poverty and hard work at part-time jobs to support his college education, his years in New York were enlivened by camaraderie with fellow-students.

He recalled practical jokes and painted a comic picture of the pedantic atmosphere of the General Theological Seminary. He graduated from Columbia in 1886, and completed his theological studies in one year, by teaching himself the first year's work over a summer and outwitting the authorities into examining him without having taken the courses. After another illness, an attack of "brain fever," Worcester decided to study philosophy and psychology in Europe, at the University of Leipzig.

When Worcester reached the University of Leipzig in 1887, this time with $100 in his pocket, he experienced the same sense of liberation and intense intellectual exhilaration that William James and G. Stanley Hall had found there, James almost twenty years before him, and Hall ten years afterward. Worcester's recollections of Leipzig are vivid, entertaining and affectionate. He believed that "a new truth dawned on me," that science was concerned not only with material things like botany and physics but with any phenomena that could be studied, classified and reduced to order. "Thus there may be a science of the immaterial and spiritual as well as the physical and material." To him this German spirit of science seemed "more liberal than ours," in removing "the false opposition" between mind and body. He found this helpful with his "later work in tuberculosis, in psychic disorders and in psychic research," the last of which meant "the gathering of evidence pointing to man's survival of bodily death."

Like other American students, Worcester had been attracted to Leipzig, rather than other European universities, by the reputation of Wilhelm Wundt, the great psychologist. He described Wundt "stealing into the great hall, attended by his *famulus*, gliding to his place on the dais." Wundt would "assume his customary position, fix his eyes on vacancy and begin to discourse," speaking for hours without notes to 600 or 800 students. Worcester took all of

Wundt's courses and seminars, but he admired Gustav Fechner even more. He regarded him as Wundt's master, in "associating the study of the mind with physics" and in establishing modern psychology as an experimental science. Indeed he wrote of Fechner, then eighty-six and in his last year of teaching, with an almost ecstatic fervor: "his soul entered so deeply into my soul, his thought so accompanied me through life, that I can no longer distinguish the transcendent quality of his mind from the man of flesh and blood."

These transcendent qualities that inspired Worcester represented the philosophical and mystical concerns that Fechner turned to in middle life, after recovering from a period of blindness. Worcester described the dramatic scene in which Fechner announced a premonition of his own death, as if he were an awe-struck witness. He wrote that Fechner's "touching words [were] engraved indelibly on the memory of all his hearers." When Worcester wrote a book about Fechner many years later, he could transcribe long passages from memory without looking up the text. Worcester later corresponded with William James, pointing out an unacknowledged source for an idea of James' in Fechner's *Three Motives*. James made a graceful reply, admitting he must have read and forgotten the passage.

In a letter to James,[6] Hall had given a very different, mildly contemptuous picture of Fechner:

[He] is a curiosity. His eyelids are strangely fringed and he has a number of holes, square and round, cut, Heaven knows why, in the iris of each eye—and is altogether a bundle of oddities in person and manner. He has forgotten all the details of his *Psychophysik;* and is chiefly interested in theorizing how knots can be tied in endless strings, and how words can be written on the inner sides of two slates sealed together. [He] wants me to go to

Zoellner and talk to him about American spiritualism, but I have not . . . [as] at present all my interest centres in *reflex action*, on which I am working with Ludwig—my first work alone.

James replied in a similar vein: "You know I always thought [Fechner's] psycho-physic as moonshiny as any of his other writings, fundamentally valuable only for its rich details." Although Fechner was eighty-six, almost ten years older when Worcester heard him lecture, Hall's and James' disdain for Fechner is a contrast with Worcester's reverence for that vatic figure. Though Fechner seems more seer and visionary than experimental scientist, both elements reflect two contrasting currents in nineteenth century thinking. The experimental trend had drawn James to Bowditch's physiology lab at Harvard Medical School in the 1870s, before establishing his own first lab in the Agassiz Museum. But despite his mockery of Fechner, James always retained his broad range of interests and his tolerance for all psychic phenomena from religious conversion to the occult.

Freud was a self-avowed admirer of Fechner, from his physiological *Project* of 1895 to his biological speculations about the death-instinct in 1920. He adapted Fechner's *Lustprinzip* for use as his "pleasure-principle," which he defined as a general regulatory principle of mental functioning, later called the "constancy principle." Freud also retained a sympathetic interest in occult phenomena, along with heterodox Lamarckian theories of evolution that Ernest Jones urged him to reject. A surprising number of other late nineteenth century scientists were interested in occult phenomena, under the guise of investigating it scientifically, as in the Society for Psychical Research. Founded in England in the 1890s, the Society was supported in this country by James, Morton Prince and Putnam, among others, and Worcester wrote about his interest in the occult throughout his life.

In the 1920s, Worcester was conducting an experimental *séance,* when the medium reported a Hamlet-like message from Worcester's own father, reproaching him for being "an undutiful son." The supposed voice of his father then revealed the existence of an unpublished geological treatise that his father had written over fifty years before, but his father's voice refused to say where it could be found. "I shall regard your willingness to search . . . as proof of your desire to serve me." When the manuscript was discovered in a forgotten trunk, it proved, according to geologists Worcester consulted, to be unusually advanced for the time it was written.

While he was at the University of Leipzig, Worcester was exposed to both experimental and metaphysical currents in modern psychology by Wundt and Fechner respectively. Despite his affinity for the visionary Fechner, he wrote his Ph.D. dissertation on the empiricist John Locke and graduated in two years. His thesis was accepted with the *censor* of *admodum laudabile,* after a traditional oral examination by the Rector Magnificus, who addressed him in Latin, "clad in a gorgeous gown and seated on a kind of throne."

When Worcester returned to the United States in 1889, his blind mother and his older sister Elizabeth, her inseparable companion, had moved from Massillon to a rooming-house in Stamford, Connecticut. His other two sisters were living in New York City, where Mary, the eldest, had become chief nurse in a large hospital and the second sister, Lina, had married a prosperous corn-broker. After a period of parish work in Brooklyn, Worcester was ordained as an Episcopal minister and applied for a post as chaplain at Lehigh University in Bethlehem, Pennsylvania.

He was accepted, and also appointed as professor of "philosophy, psychology and Christian evidences." He taught a course in each subject, and a fourth course in physical anthropology. He found teaching very enjoyable, but his sermons, at a college with compulsory chapel and many engineering students, proved to be a frustrating bore. Despite being a teetotaler, Worcester was known as a cheerful, convivial bachelor. He was warmly received by local society, and within a few years he met and married Blanche Rulison, the shy, beautiful daughter of his local bishop.

During these peaceful years in rural Pennsylvania, Worcester was surprised to find "my psychological reading turning more and more to abnormal psychology," as the clinical studies of the neuroses were then called. From Charcot and the other French neurologists, he concluded that "human nature . . . could only be understood through the knowledge of psycho-pathology." But he pursued these studies for some years without thinking they would ever have any practical value. The couple's first child, Constance, was born in 1896, and in the same year Worcester received an unexpected call to become rector of St. Stephen's in Philadelphia. This invitation followed a guest-sermon he gave during a summer vacation, substituting for his father-in-law, Bishop Rulison.

Though he enjoyed teaching, and had been offered a professorship in psychology at a larger university just before, his memoirs are brief and noncommittal about his reasons for giving up teaching and taking on the full-time duties of a pastor. He offered conventional motives: his desire to "render personal and spiritual help . . . to a more mature and diversified congregation." But his account of his next eight years at St. Stephen's, successful but uneventful, provides no deeper understanding of his decision.

Worcester's description of his Philadelphia period is lively enough, in a downtown parish that was still the most fashionable in the city, where he was popular and well-liked. Among observations about its local features, the peculiarities of Philadelphia society and some of its members, he recalled in some detail the celebrated Dr. Weir Mitchell.

Still known for the "rest-cure" treatment of neurasthenia,[7] Mitchell was also famous as a spellbinding conversationalist, for his sumptuous dinner-parties and for his many popular novels. Worcester's son and a second daughter were born in Philadelphia, and he wrote a book on Old Testament scholarship that was well-received. But there is a note of disappointment about the city, about the lack of intellectual curiosity among his parishioners, better known for their wine-cellars and terrapin suppers than their earlier Quaker traditions of radical philanthropy. Philadelphia was also the citadel of medical conservatism, opposed to the new psychotherapies of suggestion then, as it was later opposed to psychoanalysis.

Worcester's disappointment in Philadelphia may also have reflected some slackening in his own intellectual curiosity, compared to his stimulating years in Leipzig. In 1904, at the age of forty-two, he rejoiced in his invitation to become Rector of the Emmanuel Church in Boston, and he remained there for the rest of his life. He knew that Boston was considered a more stimulating city than Philadelphia, and he later reflected: "The peculiar form my ministry, all unknown to me, was to take, never could have found acceptance in Philadelphia. Boston is far more nervous than New York; Philadelphia is, or was, hardly nervous at all."

Again his parish was similar to St. Stephen's, in the recently fashionable Back Bay, slightly overshadowed by Trinity Cathedral, and again Worcester was slightly disappointed when he failed to find "the inquiring spirit" in his congregation, or indeed in the Episcopal Church itself. "I had shared the usual belief that Boston was more intellectual than other American cities. As far as the Episcopal Church is concerned, this has not been true during the last generation. None of our parishes contains any considerable group of eager seekers after truth and religious knowledge. This may be because such persons had already been satiated with Boston's innumerable lectures and were not in the habit of going to church for instruction."

In retrospect, we know that the Boston of that time was a highly mobile city, despite its reputation for social stability. Between 1880 and 1890 the population had increased 24%, and continued to grow at this rate until the 1920s. Within Boston and its suburbs there was also a continuous internal migration into and out of the city,[8] creating a much greater turn-over of population than its net growth would suggest. Although new European immigration had passed its peak in Boston by 1890, 35% of its population was foreign-born and 15% came from other states, a pattern that persisted into the 1920s.

These shifting population patterns were associated with widespread poverty, social instability and severe public health deficiencies. These problems, in turn, provided the impetus for the many social reform movements that Boston was famous for at the turn of the century. South End House was established by Robert C. Woods in 1891, shortly after Jane Addams, in Chicago, had founded Hull House, the first American settlement house. Medical social service, as an independent profession with its own training, was first introduced in the outpatient clinics of Massachusetts General Hospital in 1905, by Miss Ida Cannon and Dr. Richard C. Cabot.[9] Putnam added a social worker to the staff of the neurology service a year later, and by 1912 Cannon had organized the first one-year course in medical social service work.[10]

This new professionalism was to supersede the era of the "friendly visitor," when help had been bestowed on the poor by genteel volunteers. These were the "gray ladies" who dressed like nurses or nuns but were unpaid and had no training. Cabot had written of these pioneers that "simple friendliness" was not enough, and Cannon had insisted that "human kindness alone cannot solve tangled social problems." Nevertheless *noblesse oblige* helped create the new philanthropic professions, as the same intrepid upper-class women became the new leaders, as teachers, trustees and directors of schools. Thus any gathering of prominent Bostonians "could resolve itself into a council of social agencies."[11] Cabot proclaimed that relations between professionals and their patients must not contain "a particle of sense of shame on the one side or of condescension on the other."

But the genteel tradition in medicine lingered here and there in New England. Dr. Joseph Pratt, another stout advocate of social services, still called his social workers "friendly visitors" well into the 1920s. And Cabot's own voluminous writings are suffused with a denatured Protestant moralism that reflected its quasi-religious origins. Cabot's intense personal reactions to the poverty of his clinic patients, many of them immigrants, was one source of his need to understand their lives and families and living conditions. Another was the practical necessity of treating many of the diseases that were caused by poverty, malnutrition and crowding. Tuberculosis for example, was present in virtually epidemic proportions, and syphilis or typhus could well be called "social diseases" because of the conditions under which they flourished. There was also a new attitude toward hysteria and neurasthenia, which were recognized in all social classes and not only regarded as a privileged affliction of upper class women. Thus Pratt could approach tuberculosis quite naturally as a psychosocial problem, to be treated by sympathetic understanding and "moral re-education," as well as by food and fresh air.

There were other important events in Boston during the first decade of the twentieth century that made 1904 a significant time for Worcester to arrive. Three of these events were public lectures, which Worcester had assumed Bostonians were overly fond of. The first of these, William

James' *Varieties of Religious Experience*,[12] were given in Edinburgh in 1902, but quickly published and widely read in Boston. James welcomed all forms of psychotherapy indiscriminately, scientific, popular and religious, as part of the same "Mind Cure Movement." He wrote:

> The spread of the movement has been due to its practical fruits, and the extremely practical turn of character of the American people has never been better shown than by the fact that this, their only decidedly original contribution to the systematic philosophy of life, should be so intimately knit up with concrete therapeutics.

The second event was the series of fifteen lectures on hysteria given by Pierre Janet[13] in 1906, at the inauguration of the new Harvard Medical School, just built in the Fenway. Janet reviewed the contributions of Charcot, the French neurologists and himself on this topic, including his own claim to priority over Freud and Breuer's method of catharsis.[14] And the third event was the famous introductory lectures of Freud,[15] given in 1909 for the twentieth anniversary of Clark University in Worcester, Massachusetts.

Three influential books were published during this same period. The first was Havelock Ellis's *Studies in the Psychology of Sex*,[16] which was an important landmark in the public acceptance of sexuality. Ironically, Ellis's six original volumes were published in conservative Philadelphia, to avoid legal problems with British censorship. They also contained a sympathetic consideration of Freud's early theories, with extensive quotations. A second book, G. Stanley Hall's *Adolescence*,[17] also furthered the public discussion of sex and reflected an earlier American interest in childhood development. A third book, *The Psychic Treatment of Nervous Disorders*,[18] by the Swiss neurologist Dubois, translated by Smith

Ely Jelliffe and William A. White in 1908, was influential as a handbook of the new psychologies of suggestion. Finally, an important journal was published in Boston, *The Journal of Abnormal Psychology*, founded by Morton Prince in 1906. Its first issue contained the first report in English on psychoanalytic treatment: James Jackson Putnam's "Recent Experiences in the Study and Treatment of Hysteria at the Massachusetts General Hospital; with remarks on Freud's Method of Treatment by 'Psycho-analysis'."[19]

Another feature that distinguished *fin-de-siècle* Boston from other American cities was the "Mother Church" of Christian Science, which was founded here and grew rapidly. Between 1892 and 1910 its membership increased by 100,000, illustrated by its monuments still visible today. The gaunt Original Edifice was built in 1894, overshadowed by the swelling neo-baroque cupola of its new church, looming over Symphony Hall. The phenomenal growth of Christian Science was a response to the same increased need for treatment of the common neuroses that nourished the new psychotherapies of suggestion. Its aggressively antimedical doctrines intensified the antagonism of local physicians toward lay-psychotherapy in any form, but in attacking Christian Science local physicians were also drawn to the support of "medical psychotherapy."[20]

In a longer historical perspective, of course, the psychotherapies of suggestion, Freudian psychoanalysis and Christian Science healing can all be seen as descendants of Anton Mesmer. They are linked together by Mrs. Eddy's famous hypnotic cure, ironically first performed by a physician, Dr. Phineas P. Quimby, and by Freud's visit to Charcot and Bernheim in the 1880s. But in the battles over licensure in the early 1890s, between Boston physicians and lay healers, only William James recognized the common denominator, "that the therapeutic relation may be what we can only at present describe as a relation of one person to another person."[21] Most physicians took an opposite view, like Cabot who claimed that Christian Science had delayed American acceptance of the new psychotherapy by ten to twenty years.

3

The New England Tradition of "Medical Psychotherapy" and its Turn-of-the-Century Practitioners

R ichard C. Cabot deplored Christian Science and faith healing in all its forms, but he welcomed the new psychotherapies of suggestion, and he became a leader among the prominent Boston physicians who practiced what I have called "medical psychotherapy." This local tradition included internists like Cabot and Joseph Pratt, neurologists like James Jackson Putnam and Morton Prince, and academic psychologists like William James, Josiah Royce and Boris Sidis. This last group, the psychologists, were not known as practicing physicians but several of them, like James and Sidis, happened to have M.D. degrees as well as the Ph.D. In its broadest sense, then, medical psychotherapy belonged to the ancient traditions of general medicine, in which the physician treated all illnesses, mental and physical. He used his intuitive understanding of his patient's personality, as well as his scientific knowledge of medicine. In a more specialized sense, medical psychotherapy meant what was practiced by late nineteenth century New England physicians who had taught themselves hypnosis and other forms of suggestion.

This was a time, as we have seen, when psychiatrists were few, and most of them were engaged in the custodial care of institutionalized psychotic patients. The majority of patients with neurotic symptoms were treated by various forms of medical psychotherapy, in private offices and outpatient clinics, rather than private asylums or state mental hospitals. Some biographical sketches of these early practitioners will illustrate the complexities of the medical scene.

Frederick H. Gerrish (1845–1920)

According to Lawrence Kubie[1], Gerrish was the first in a line of development that reached its fullest expression in the Austen Riggs Foundation at Stockbridge, Massachusetts. As a surgeon in Portland, Maine, Gerrish was already practicing "a Down East version of French psychotherapy-through-suggestion" in the early 1880s. Born in Portland and educated at Bowdoin, he took his medical degree in 1869. His first interest was microscopy, which he studied in New York City, and he returned to Maine as a lecturer in materia medica, therapeutics and physiology. He wrote many papers on public health and rural medicine, a report on the sewage and water-supply of Portland, and a popular handbook on prescription-writing. By 1880 he had become a convert to "Listerism," as well as a practicing general surgeon. During this decade he was president of the American Academy of Medicine and director of the Maine Board of Health. He began to edit *A Textbook of Anatomy by American Authors,* two-thirds of which he wrote himself.

When and how Gerrish became a passionate advocate of hypnosis is hard to establish. Kubie's researches suggest that he had studied abroad with Bernheim, Dubois and

Charcot, but Curran[2] found no evidence for this. In 1892, Gerrish published an enthusiastic paper on the applications of hypnosis to surgery, medicine and psychotherapy. He referred to writings of the French neurologists, and reported that he had used hypnosis almost daily in a year's practice, "which now covers about 1500 applications." Until his retirement in 1911, he was professor of both anatomy and surgery at Bowdoin Medical College, and he continued to lecture on medical ethics until his death in 1920.

As president of the American Therapeutic Society in 1908, Gerrish became a leader among medical advocates of "modern" psychotherapy, meaning hypnosis and suggestion. For its annual meeting in May 1909, Gerrish organized a remarkable symposium on the treatment of the neuroses, with the advice and collaboration of Morton Prince. All the important figures in the psychotherapy movement were represented, a majority from Boston, and the proceedings were published in a small book, called simply *Psychotherapeutics*.[3] Prince gave a rousing keynote address, reviewing the scope of the field in an optimistic vein. Gerrish spoke on the applications of hypnotic suggestion in surgery and medicine, and Sidis lectured on "the hypnoidal state" in hysteria. Putnam's paper acknowledged the contributions of Janet, Bergson and Freud, and gave an accurate, somewhat euphemistic account of Freud's theories about the sexual etiology of hysteria.

Another speaker, Ernest Jones, who was living in Toronto at that time and thus became a temporary "American," was very active in American scientific life and considered himself already an advocate for psychoanalysis. With a confident sense of his general medical audience, Jones gave a skillful popularization of psychoanalysis as "the second stage in the evolution of psychotherapy." He differentiated the suggestive methods of hypnosis from the psychoanalytic methods of free-association, comparing the latter to the "draining of a tubercular, or better still of an actinomycotic abscess." He contrasted the "orthopedic straightening of a deformed limb" with the "far more intricate task of the orthopsychic training of a deformed mind." Jones acknowledged that Freud required as much as an hour a day for three years to treat difficult cases, but, he suggested reassuringly, "in milder cases one can achieve very satisfactory results in a few months, a fact to which I can fully attest from my own experience."[4]

This meeting took place in New Haven, five months before the far better known Clark University meeting at Worcester, where Freud gave his now famous introductory lectures on psychoanalysis. But the proceedings of the American Therapeutic Society gives us a vivid glimpse of an interesting transitional phase, when the "new" psychotherapy was still at its peak of popularity, and psychoanalysis was seen as an even newer variant from abroad.

Gerrish himself was an energetic, self-taught enthusiast, with strong interests in many different fields, from sewage-systems to hypnosis. Even a brief biography suggests the kind of quirky, eccentric figure that is familiar in nineteenth century American medicine. His biographer in the *Dictionary of American Biography*[5] calls him "an unusual but rather disharmonic personality," a stickler for precision, feared by his anatomy-students, but witty and humorous. He was an agnostic with "an almost spinsterish aversion to certain foibles and petty vices," an idealist about education and public health, and an advocate of simplified spelling and "marital continence save for procreation."

John George Gehring (1857–1932)

Gerrish's dramatic cure of George Gehring by hypnosis was the impetus that led Gehring to create a treatment-center for neuroses that was the model for Austen Riggs and other private sanitaria. But the accidental encounter between the two men was part of a complex sequence of coincidences, going back to President McKinley's assassination and the famous surgeon, Charles McBurney, of the anatomical landmark "McBurney's Point."

McBurney was a classmate of Austen Riggs' father[6], a physician who had died early of tuberculosis. McBurney became a family adviser to the young widow, and virtually a father to Austen, who eventually married McBurney's daughter. When the young Austen Riggs was himself convalescing from tuberculosis, the elderly McBurney was being treated at Gehring's sanitarium at Bethel, Maine, for some unnamed nervous condition. Riggs visited him at Bethel, sometime in 1908, and wrote his mother enthusiastically about the atmosphere, Gehring's personality and his philosophy of treatment for "those cases that occupied the No Man's Land between medicine and psychiatry." Riggs was impressed by the improvement in an aunt of his who was being treated at Bethel, by the outdoor regimen for all patients, and by the celebrated daily stint of manual labor at the woodpile.

From this experience, and his readings in the works of the French neurologists, of William James and of Breuer and Freud, Riggs evolved his own form of "medical psychotherapy." By 1913 he had established a residential treatment-center for the neuroses, very similar to Gehring's at Bethel, with its program of compulsory "work-therapy" outdoors. Riggs' unusual personality sustained this unique institution, which became the Austen Riggs Foundation at Stockbridge, Massachusetts. It survived in its original form long enough to undergo a dramatic transformation in the early 1950s, with the arrival of Robert P. Knight, Erik Erikson, David Rapaport and other eminent psychoanalysts from the Menninger Foundation. Thus Austen Riggs, through his encounter with Gehring, had become the consummate medical psychotherapist, without ever having studied clinical psychiatry, and created a link with the psychoanalytic tradition of a later day.

Returning to the life of John George Gehring, he was born in Cleveland, studied medicine at Western Reserve and graduated in 1885. He was twenty-eight, somewhat older than most medical students of that period. Like Gerrish, Gehring became a surgeon and practiced in Cleveland until some acute emotional disturbance caused him to leave that city. Myths and speculations proliferated about Gehring's disappearance, according to Kubie: a dramatic flight in the midst of an operation, or a secret addiction to one of the new anesthetic agents. By 1887 Gehring had settled in the remote village of Bethel, in northeastern Maine, where he farmed, lived in seclusion and married a recent widow. According to some of Kubie's informants, Gehring continued to have emotional crises, for which he consulted Gerrish in Portland. According to another source[7], he was seeking treatment for his wife, who had once been a patient of Weir Mitchell in Philadelphia. When the Gehrings were on their way to Philadelphia by train, Mrs. Gehring became so acutely ill that they were forced to stop at Portland, where they reached Gerrish's office entirely by accident. Dr. Gerrish proved "so successful in his psychotherapy that Mrs. Gehring refused to go on to Philadelphia." Gehring, who was suffering from a similar emotional disturbance, also became Gerrish's patient, and both improved rapidly within a few weeks. Gehring "returned to Bethel a convert, and with missionary zeal set out to convince the local doctors . . . of this new form of treatment."

The Gehrings' dramatic cure occurred between 1893 and 1895, within the first years of Gerrish's "conversion" to the practice of hypnosis. Gehring had studied at the University of Berlin in 1891, and not, as Kubie assumed, after graduating from medical school. He later took many trips to

Europe with his wife, and once visited Bernheim at Nancy,[8] as Prince, Freud and many other physicians had done. By 1895, at any rate, Gehring was successfully treating patients at Bethel with Gerrish's hypnotic methods. At first his patients stayed in his house, and later at the Prospect Hotel. When this burned down in 1912, the Bethel Inn was built as a testimonial by a group of his grateful patients. Some came for short or repeated visits, others for months or years. A few settled in Bethel, like the wealthy philanthropist, William Bingham, who spent part of each year there, from 1911 until his death in 1955.

Gehring's therapeutic methods included a systematic regime of group living, with a schedule of meals together, outdoor work-periods and athletics. His patients met for dinner in formal dress, followed by an evening of lectures, amateur theatrical performances or lantern-slides. In his individual psychotherapy, Gehring emphasized the value of a complete "talking out," which he began by spending several hours with each patient, with shorter visits on successive days, to enable his patient to "tell his whole story in one piece."[9] Apparently the patient lay on a couch, while Gehring sat behind the patient, making use of some hypnosis and "waking suggestion" as needed. Writing about his methods in 1923, Gehring emphasized the unity of mind and body and the futility of reason and logical persuasion:

> in order that such measures shall succeed, they must sink in upon the subconsciousness, and that is often a slow and trying process since the consciousness must first be appeased. Doubtless, often when we have succeeded, it will be because we have effected a direct subconscious entrance without our knowing it.[10]

These commonsense approaches reflected some awareness of Freudian theory, but they were expressed in the pre-analytic language of Morton Prince (*subconscious* instead of *unconscious*, etc.). Although Gehring sometimes referred to his method as "a form of psychoanalysis," Kubie pointed out that Gehring "seems to have had no inkling of the role of transference in producing transitory therapeutic results." Nevertheless Gehring made intuitive use of his forceful personality to influence symptoms, as vividly portrayed in Robert Herrick's romanticized novel about Bethel[11] and in the memoirs of Max Eastman.[12] Gehring had diagnosed Eastman as a case of "imperfect nerve-tissue, which all Brahmins have," and talked away his symptoms in a "gruff, friendly voice [that] 'suggested' tranquillity and fortitude rather than health." This pattern recalls the methods of many famous "healers," who attributed their results to some formal regimen rather than the force of their own personalities.

Robert T. Edes (1838–1923)

As an exemplar of medical psychotherapy, Edes was one of the first in Boston, and best known for his 1895 Shattuck Lectures, "The New England Invalid."[13] In this three-part address to the Massachusetts Medical Society, Edes exhorted *all* physicians to recognize and treat the nervous symptoms of their patients, especially those presenting as bodily complaints. He referred to George Beard's belief that "nervousness has been called the American disease," and quoted a description by a Dr. Loewenfeld of Munich about urban crowding and economic competition as causes of nervous tension. But, Edes asked, "Is not the disposing cause the spirit of the times and not the spirit of the country?" Then he quoted Miss Catherine Beecher, the pioneer feminist, writing forty years before his time: "I cannot recall, in my immense circle of friends and acquaintances all over the Union, more than ten married ladies . . . who are perfectly sound, healthy and vigorous."

From among her own nine married sisters and sisters-in-law (including Mrs. Harriet Beecher Stowe), and her four-teen female cousins, Miss Beecher recalled only two women who were "not either delicate, often ailing or an invalid."[14]

Edes expressed doubts about the importance of both hereditary and climatic factors, at a time when they were still prevailing medical beliefs, especially in Europe. Instead, he asserted, "habits of thought are largely formed and modified in childhood." He classified 1,000 of his own patients, in a busy medical practice, as follows: melancholia 97 patients, neurasthenia 490, hysteria 197 and hypochondriasis 33. He doubted that American patients show "the fully developed hysteria of the Salpêtrière . . . The American neurologist must content himself with fewer and less picturesque cases." Then he offered his own subtypes, including the Malingerer, the Tense Neurasthenic and the Limp Neurasthenic. He concluded that he had never seen an authentic case of malingering, in the sense of consciously feigning illness.

Among some lively and anecdotal case-histories, he referred to recent studies by Breuer and Freud on the treatment of hysteria by the "cathartic method." Although he spoke favorably of their results, he concluded that they are "not far removed from the commonsense observation that it is much better to 'get mad' and be done with it than to cherish the grievance in silence. The effort of inhibition seems to call for as much expenditure of energy as action . . . and of that peculiarly unremitting and wearing character which is so silently destructive of nervous integrity. There should be a proper balance between the inflow of irritations and the outflow of nervous energy."

Edes dismissed current medical beliefs that some inherent weakness in women was a cause of neurosis, quoting Dr. Mary Putnam Jacobi to the effect that menstrual disorders were more likely to be the result of nervousness than its cause. He was skeptical about other fashionable theories suggesting an etiological role for auto-intoxication, anemia or malnutrition. The last of these conditions was the rationale for Weir Mitchell's well-known "rest-cure," which combined overfeeding with total inactivity.

Edes concluded his lectures with some observant and highly critical comments on his medical colleagues' reactions to their patients with nervous disorders. He sympathized with his fellow-physicians' helpless frustration at being unable to help their patients, and with their defensive anger and disdain for nervous disorders. But he noted their tendency to refer neurotic patients to other doctors and deplored their desperate recourse to placebos of all kinds, especially the use of deceitful and dangerous sham-operations. The methods of treatment he advised instead were the commonsense ones of that era, including rest and healthful activity. But Edes' real message to his colleagues, as we understand it today, was his emphasis on listening to their patients' symptoms, bringing some scientific curiosity about their meaning, and above all taking their complaints seriously, as painful and disabling conditions.

This essentially humane and commonsense approach to neurotic invalidism foreshadowed James Jackson Putnam's Shattuck Lecture four years later.[15] Putnam's address was a far more impassioned plea to the general physician, urging him to concern himself with the individual personality and life-situation of his patients. Putnam acknowledged the inadequacy of current therapeutic measures, and called for changes in medical education that would improve the understanding of neuroses. Both Edes and Putnam were addressing all physicians, not specialists in neurology or psychopathology, and thus helped to define a tradition of medical psychotherapy. In this tradition every physician was his own psychiatrist, without using that term, which was then usually reserved for the "alienist" in a state asylum. Its methods of treatment were derived from Charcot and Bernheim, DuBois and Déjérine, the same methods that were used by neurologists like Morton Prince and E. W. Taylor.

Edes was born in 1838 at Eastport, Maine, the son of a Unitarian minister, whose father sent him to Harvard. He graduated from Harvard College and from Harvard Medical School in 1861, when he joined the Navy and had an active career as a surgeon during the Civil War. He returned to Boston after the war, practiced medicine and taught at Harvard Medical School and Boston City Hospital. He became James Jackson Professor of Clinical Medicine in 1884, a distinguished chair named for James Jackson Putnam's grandfather. Two years later he suddenly resigned, "because of illness in the family,"[16] and moved to Washington D.C. There he lectured at Georgetown and other local medical schools, and wrote a textbook of therapeutics and materia medica.

Five years later he returned to Boston and became superintendent of Dr. Adams' Nervine Asylum in Jamaica Plain, adjoining the Arnold Arboretum. "The Nervine," as it was fondly called by old Boston families, was another remarkable residential center for the treatment of the neuroses, very much like the sanitaria of Gehring at Bethel and Riggs at Stockbridge. Here Edes was able to practice the kind of medical psychotherapy he had advocated in his Shattuck lectures, although the Adams Nervine later became a more conventional private mental hospital. Its stately buildings were taken over by the adjoining Faulkner Hospital, and recently were converted into condominiums, skillfully preserving their original nineteenth century elegance.

After six years, Edes once again retired from his position as superintendent and moved to Springfield, when he became depressed following the death of a gifted young son, at the age of thirty-two. He gave up the practice of medicine, but he continued to write for the local papers and died at eighty-five in 1923. He had written two novels, the first based on his Civil War experiences, *The Story of Rodman Heath; or, Mugwumps by One of Them*, and the second about the French and Indian Wars, *Parson Gay's Three Sermons; or Saint Sacremont*.

Thus Edes seemed to become a medical psychotherapist through his clinical experiences as a surgeon and internist, and possibly also, like other contemporary Americans, he was drawn to "abnormal psychology," by some personal encounter with mental illness in himself or his family. Edes, like Riggs, became what we would now call psychiatrists, while Cabot and Pratt remained general physicians who also practiced psychotherapy.

George M. Beard, Boris Sidis and Henry Linenthal

Before concluding this chapter on medical psychotherapy with biographical sketches of Richard Cabot and Joseph Pratt, who played important parts in the Emmanuel Movement, a few other practitioners of medical psychotherapy can be described more briefly. George M. Beard (1839–1883), already mentioned for introducing the term "neurasthenia" and the concept of "American Nervousness," could be considered an outstanding example of the New England psychotherapy tradition, although he was born in Connecticut, attended Yale and settled in New York.[17] He also favored treatment with galvanic electricity ("faradism") rather than the hypnosis and suggestion of his Boston colleagues. Like Edes, he was the son of a Congregational minister, born in 1839. After graduating from Yale, he attended the Medical College of Physicians & Surgeons in New York, and received his M.D. degree in 1866. But even as a medical student he had served as acting assistant surgeon in the Navy during the Civil War, and he published his first paper in 1866, "Electricity as a Tonic."

Beard continued to explore the medical uses of low-voltage galvanic current, and wrote papers that became popular among German neurologists, which gave him some international renown. (By coincidence, Freud's discouragement with the electrical treatment of hysterical conversion symptoms led him to explore the French neurologists' use of hypnosis.) From Beard's medical school master's thesis, "The Longevity of Brain-Workers,"[18] he pursued the idea that Americans suffered from more nervous disorders than other nationalities, especially "nervous exhaustion," or "neurasthenia," which he defined as a depletion of "nerve force." He attributed American susceptibility to neurosis as a result of *modern civilization*, "which is distinguished from the ancient by these five characteristics: steam-power, the periodical press, the telegraph, the sciences and the mental activity of women." To these he added secondary and tertiary causes: the American climate, "dryness of the air, extremes of heat and cold, civil and religious liberty and the great mental activity" required to be productive under such climatic conditions.[19]

He was a prolific writer, from popular books like *Our Home Physician* (1869) to his best known *Nervous Exhaustion* (1880). He was a lecturer on nervous diseases at New York University, and gave papers at international meetings. He also wrote about sea-sickness, the Salem witch-trials and problems of aging. After the assassination of President Garfield, he defended the unpopular position that Guiteau was insane and not legally responsible. He died in 1883, relatively young, regretting the fact that he could not record his dying thoughts but hoping others would continue his work.

Boris Sidis (1867–1923) occupied an unusual position in the tradition of medical psychotherapy, because he began among the clinical psychologists like William James and later became a physician practicing the psychotherapy of suggestion. Sidis' reputation for early brilliance and originality was achieved as a student of James and Hugo Münsterberg. As a Russian immigrant, he entered Harvard College in 1892, completed his bachelor's degree in two years and obtained both his M.A. and Ph.D. degrees in 1897. He published his first book the same year, *The Psychology of Suggestion*,[20] and moved to New York, where he worked in the New York State hospital system, under both Adolf Meyer and William A. White. Although Manhattan State, on Welfare Island, had been an early source of enthusiasm for Freudian theories during Meyer's era,[21] Sidis became highly critical of psychoanalysis. He developed his own theories about hysteria, based on the "hypnoid state," and his own version of psychotherapy by suggestion.

He returned to Boston, entered Harvard Medical School, and graduated in 1908. He later established his own Psychotherapeutic Institute in Portsmouth, New Hampshire. In 1909 he took part in Gerrish's symposium on the treatment of nervous disorders, where he argued against the analytic theories of Putnam and Ernest Jones. He published books and papers during the high tide of the psychotherapy movement, but during his later years in Portsmouth he was no longer prominent in the Boston scientific scene.

Harry Linenthal (1876–1954) also forms an interesting link between the psychotherapies of suggestion and the early writings of Freud, which he had read as a medical student and translated for Putnam and Morton Prince.[22] Like Sidis, he was born in Russia and emigrated to Boston with his family in 1891. Lacking formal schooling, he worked by day and studied English and other subjects in the evening. His tutor, in fact, happened to be Boris Sidis himself, who had arrived in Boston in 1887, and tutored fellow immigrants in order to work his way through school. Linenthal completed four years of high school, graduated with honors from Harvard College and earned his M.D. degree from Harvard in 1904. During this process he became a close friend of Sidis, who had returned to Boston and completed his own medical training only four years later than his pupil.

Through his association with Sidis, Linenthal became enthusiastic about the new treatment of neurosis by suggestion. Because he was unable, as a Jew, to obtain a staff appointment at the Massachusetts General Hospital,[23] he worked there as a "voluntary assistant," without pay, in the out-patient Neurology Clinic under Putnam. This was the period when Putnam was experimenting with the treatment of hysteria and other neuroses in the clinic. After encountering some staff resistance, Putnam finally obtained two beds on the dermatology service! Putnam was also experimenting with his own version of "Breuer and Freud's Cathartic Method," which he reported in his landmark paper of 1906.[24] What Putnam called "psychoanalysis" was not what psychoanalysis became in later years, as Hale,[25] Burnham[26] and Taylor[27] have pointed out, but his 1906 paper still deserves acclaim as a first significant step in the acceptance of analysis by the American public, as it was regarded by Freud.

In 1904, the year Linenthal graduated from medical school, he published with others a paper[28] reporting the same kind of cases as Putnam's. This paper reflected the characteristically ambiguous position that Freudian theories occupied during the high tide of the psychotherapy movement. One of the cases reported, treated in the Massachusetts General Hospital out-patient neurology clinic, was a young Russian immigrant like Linenthal himself, who had suffered "attacks" of hemianesthesia and epileptiform jerking movements for five years. The authors paid homage to "Breuer and Freud's classic work, which has helped to change our conception of the disease [hysteria]," but their psychodynamic formulation in terms of "dissociation" more closely resembled the theories of Janet and the

French school. The cure, over a period of weekly visits, was accomplished by hypnotic regression to the age when the original trauma occurred, and by making the patient recall these events in the waking state. "The subconscious and the waking memories are thus united," the authors concluded. They called their method "treatment by association," which contained elements of both suggestive psychotherapy and psychoanalysis, without using the term "repression." Their summary clearly illustrated how Freudian theories were seen as one of the suggestive therapies, when they compared their case to those "studied by Janet in France, Breuer and Freud in Germany [sic], and a number of cases studied in this country by Sidis and Prince."

Linenthal's collaborator, E. W. Taylor, had been a student of Putnam and became an eminent neurologist, but, like Sidis, he later grew antagonistic toward psychoanalysis. But at that time when distinctions were less sharply drawn, Linenthal continued to treat patients with neuroses at the Massachusetts General Hospital. In another paper,[29] he described a young woman with recurrent hysterical aphonia, related to a consciously withheld secret. She was cured by being persuaded to reveal her secret, and by interpreting to her its relationship to her symptom. Freud is referred to for having "pointed out the important role which *suppressed* mental states play in the activities of our daily life" [italics added]. Thus, Linenthal wrote that "an unpleasant emotional experience" is suppressed and "will discharge itself in an abnormal path . . .'converted' into a somatic phenomenon." In this, and another case, the authors make some use of Freud's concept of hysterical conversion, but apply it to conscious events which are "suppressed" and the patient can be reasoned into accepting.

Linenthal translated and abstracted several volumes of Janet for Morton Prince, and contributed abstracts and articles on psychotherapy to Prince's *Journal of Abnormal Psy-*

chology. Even after Linenthal had left the Massachusetts General Hospital clinic in 1907, to accept a position with the State Board of Health, he retained his interest in the treatment of the neuroses. In 1909, he was strongly recommended for the directorship of the new Juvenile Psychopathic Institute in Chicago, later the Institute for Juvenile Research. Linenthal's growing interest in public health and preventive medicine led him to decline this position, which was taken by William Healy, who in 1917 became the director of the Judge Baker Guidance Center in Boston.

In 1913 Linenthal was appointed to the staff of the Massachusetts General Hospital, the first Jewish physician to break through a traditional but unacknowledged anti-Semitic barrier. This was the result of determined efforts by Richard Cabot, then chief of the West Medical Service. He had admired Linenthal during their years in the out-patient clinics, and he was indignant that the Massachusetts General Hospital "had gone for 101 years without a single Jewish physician."[30] The rest of Linenthal's career is interesting in itself for his pioneer forays in public health. He investigated tuberculosis control, ophthalmia neonatorum, lead poisoning and the widespread hazards in the sweatshops and crowded, unhealthy housing of the immigrant poor, the same "psychosocial" conditions that concerned Cabot and Pratt. Although Linenthal's scientific interests turned away from psychiatry, he continued to treat patients with "medical psychotherapy" in his private practice. He made a conscious effort to remain a generalist, a "family physician" rather than either an internist or a psychiatrist, still delivering babies and treating hysterical conversion symptoms. As physician-in-chief at Beth Israel Hospital until 1946, his interests contributed to the warm reception encountered by the first refugee physicians and psychoanalysts from Nazi Germany and Austria in the 1930s.

Richard C. Cabot (1868–1939)

Cabot was a prominent representative of medical psycho-therapy, well-known among internists but best remembered among psychiatrists and social workers because he was the first to establish a medical social service department at the Massachusetts General Hospital in 1905. He came from an ancient, complex Boston family like Putnam's, in which Putnam's wife, for example, was a Cabot from a different branch of the family. There was a strong philanthropic tradition that created physicians, philosophers and social reformers, and sometimes all three at once. His father was an architect, philosopher and biographer of Emerson; his cousin, Joseph Lee, devoted his life to social work and the settlement-house movement; and his wife, Ella Lyman Cabot, was a well-known teacher and writer on ethics and educational psychology.

As a promising young internist at the turn of the century, Cabot was a gifted teacher and the author of many text-books on physical diagnosis, heart-disease and the blood. His career at the Massachusetts General Hospital, where he became chief of medicine in 1912, had interrelations with Putnam, Linenthal and later with Worcester. His interest in social work seemed to arise from a sense of therapeutic helplessness that confronted him when he encountered the many poor and foreign-born patients who filled the wards and the new out-patient clinics. He recruited nurses, as he had recruited his first social worker, Garnet Pelton. He sought the support of Putnam who shared his concerns, and collaborated with Ida Cannon from 1907 onward.[31] In many papers, Cabot[32] described the overwhelming impression that the immigrant population made on him. Their poverty, malnutrition, physical illness and emotional suffering, Cabot wrote, led him to seek information about each patient's "home, his work, his family, his worries . . . Facing my own failures day after day, my work came to seem almost intolerable."

These encounters with the poor, besides stirring his interest in social work, made Cabot an early advocate of pre-paid medical care in his efforts to change both society and the medical profession. In 1913 he was almost expelled from the Massachusetts Medical Society for his radical views on current medical practices, specifically for "publicly advertising the faults of the general physician." In 1920 he became the first professor of Social Ethics at Harvard, and he wrote books about ethics, religion, pastoral counseling and psychotherapy. Once influential but almost unreadable today, they are redolent with that mixture of self-improvement, optimism and dilute Christianity that characterized so many well-intentioned products of New England Protestantism.

Coming from this background, Cabot soon became a supporter of the Emmanuel Movement, with its combined appeal to patients with tuberculosis and nervous disorders. With his usual enthusiasm, Cabot wrote to defend Dr. Worcester against the attacks of organized medicine. Putnam had also been an initial supporter, and before the first group-meeting in Emmanuel Church, he had asked Cabot to give the introductory lecture to the "Neurasthenic Class," as the group of patients was called. By 1908, Putnam[33] had become critical of the Emmanuel Movement, but Cabot continued to defend it vigorously. He asked Putnam what "mistake" of Worcester's he had heard about: "Have you known or heard of any other cases in which you think harm can reasonably be attributed to the Emmanuel work?" Even if there had been, Cabot continued,[34] occasional harm was no reason to stop work; he and Putnam, he acknowledged, had occasionally harmed a patient, but generally "we do little harm and considerable good. Worcester on the whole seems to me to do as much good as any physician I know and so far—until your letter—I have heard of no harm."

Besides his personal confidence in Worcester, Cabot had a general preference for the amateur over the medical expert in dealing with emotional problems, just as Pratt later considered general practitioners better suited for treating neurotic patients than psychiatrists. In a 1911 letter to Putnam,[35] Cabot assailed psychoanalysis on similar grounds, for its narrow medical specialization, for "paddling in the shallows of a huge ocean" whose depths have been better explored by social workers, novelists like Meredith and Chesterton, by Swedenborg, and by Cardinal Newman, an unusual set of bed-fellows.

4

Joseph Hersey Pratt and the Origins of Group-Therapy

Our last exemplar of the medical psychotherapy tradition, Joseph H. Pratt (1872–1956), was the starting-point of the Emmanuel Movement, as the first to use the group meetings that became a distinctive feature of Worcester's method of treatment. Like Cabot, Pratt had received the very best medical training of his time and was always known as an internist and clinician. Many decades later he was called "the father of group psychotherapy," in Slavson's history of the movement,[1] but these admiring references to his priority often failed to distinguish between two phases in Pratt's career. The first, from which the Emmanuel Movement evolved, began in 1905 when Pratt devised his "class method" for the treatment of tuberculosis. Worcester was his assistant, and their meetings took place in the Emmanuel Church. The second, separated by several decades, began in the 1930s, when Pratt opened his "Thought-Control Clinic" at the Medical Clinic of the Boston Dispensary. These groups met for the treatment of neuroses and functional disorders (not tuberculosis), referred from the Dispensary's medical out-patients.

Although most medical historians agree that Pratt deserved credit for being the first group therapist, as the creator of his original tuberculosis "classes," there were other pioneers of group psychotherapy between 1905 and 1930. First among them was, of course, Pratt's collaborator and ally, the Rev. Elwood Worcester, who had adapted Pratt's tuberculosis classes to the treatment of nervous disorders in 1906. Pratt contributed to this confusion about priorities by later disclaiming any connection with "the so-called 'Emmanuel Movement' for the treatment of nervous disorders,[2]" and in 1953 he repeated this statement to an historian of the group-therapy movement.[3]

Without attempting a full history of group-psychotherapy, a few of these early experimenters with group-methods will be briefly described, in order to clarify Pratt's originality. The large number of these pioneers is significant in itself, and most of them were unaware of Pratt's or anyone else's group experiments, as if early twentieth century America had provided the ideal soil for the self-germination of group-treatment. Hadden[4] illustrates the phenomenon, in seeming to be unaware of Pratt's or Worcester's work and basing his 1930 group-treatment of neuroses on methods used for treating tuberculosis by Joseph Walsh in 1923. In the histories previously mentioned by Slavson and Rosenbaum, the earliest group practitioner after Worcester was M. L. Cody,[5] also a clergyman, who treated neuroses in 1909–1914 and may have been influenced by the Emmanuel Movement. Trigant Burrow[6] was a founding member of the American Psychoanalytic Association in 1911, and used group-methods in the early 1920s, but he worked in relative isolation from both fellow analysts and other group-psychotherapists. Lazell[7] may have treated schizophrenia with group-methods even earlier at St. Elizabeth's, with the encouragement of William A. White, but his work belongs to the expansive period in group therapy after 1930, along with the work of Slavson, Schilder and others.

All of these early group-therapists were American except for Paul Schilder (1886–1940), a Viennese whose enthusiasm for a form of "analytic group-psychotherapy" emerged only after he emigrated to the US and settled in New York in 1931. Even J. L. Moreno (1892–1974), the creator of "psycho-drama," who dated the origins of "scientific group therapy" to 1931, claimed that "the child [of group therapy] was conceived in Vienna, but it was born in America.[8]" He traced its origins to his experiments as a story-teller with groups of children in the parks of Vienna around 1910, which he continued with prostitutes in the Viennese red-light district, *Am Spittelberg.* His claims were sweeping, tracing pre-scientific group therapy back to primitive relig-ious rituals and even the origins of multicellular organisms. He emphasized the opposition between psychoanalysis and group psychotherapy, the individual vs. the group, even though so many later group therapists were analysts or strongly influenced by analysis. Moreno dismissed Pratt's pioneering status as a myth, and called his "class method" of treating tuberculosis patients in 1905 mere "lectures . . . to give them information about a hygienic regimen."

Joseph H. Pratt (1872–1956)

Joseph Hersey Pratt was born in Middleborough, Massa-chusetts in 1872, and educated at Yale and Johns Hopkins under William Osler. He spent four years of research on pathology at Boston City Hospital, and studied at Rudolf Krehl's clinic in Tübingen. Returning to Boston from Ger-many in 1902, he began to practice internal medicine, while devoting part of each day to laboratory or clinical research. He was appointed to the medical clinics of the Massachusetts General Hospital and remained an instructor at Harvard until 1917. Ten years later he became professor of medicine at Tufts Medical School and chief of the Boston Dispensary. He had developed a pioneer program for rural medicine in 1931, and wrote over a hundred papers, a textbook of physical diagnosis and a memoir about his studies with Osler.

Like Cabot, Pratt's concern with the emotional and sociological aspects of illness arose during his first years at the Massachusetts General Hospital, treating outpatients with all the problems of poverty and social disorganization. He was appalled by the numbers of patients with tuberculosis, several hundred a year, sometimes two to three new cases each morning, and especially by those who were unable to pay for the required sanitarium treatment. Some could not afford the small weekly charge for the State sanitarium at Rutland, some were rejected for sanitarium care because of advanced and presumably incurable disease, and others could not afford to stop working, in order to support their families.

Pratt's ideas for the "outdoor treatment" of tuberculosis evolved from an encounter with two typical young women, sisters who had come to the clinic together. The elder sister presented with an advanced case, and the younger with tuberculosis in its early stages. Pratt advised the younger that her sister's prognosis was poor, but that her own infection could be arrested by sanitarium care. For the younger sister this was impossible, because her work was necessary to support her sister and their invalid parents. Disturbed by his inability to help these patients, and others like them, Pratt consulted the Rev. Worcester, newly arrived in Boston and looking for a socially useful project. From this meeting of the two men, the first Emmanuel Church Tuberculosis Class was held in July 1905.

The "class method" was also a method of treating patients at home, instead of in sanitaria, and its first optimistic results had been reported in 1905, in a periodical with the delightful name of *Journal of the Outdoor Life*,[9] and later in more conventional medical journals.[10] The "outdoor" element in the treatment was a dramatic example of the "fresh air movement," among many zealous nineteenth century efforts to promote the medical benefits of fresh air. Its origins go back to the idealization of nature in early Romanticism, the cult of sports, physical exercise and long walks in the country, and the treatment of tuberculosis by "healthful surroundings." Its local effects can still be recognized in the original Peter Bent Brigham Hospital, which was built in 1909, with its widely spaced pavilions and open-air passageways, seemingly modeled on the plans for a Swiss tuberculosis sanitarium. The hospital's outpatient clinics were still called "The Outdoor Department" until the late 1940s. The open-air classrooms at the Shady Hill School in Cambridge, founded by two famous Harvard professors, W. E. Hocking and George Sarton, with its chilly regimen of reciting outdoors, is within living memory.[11]

The class-method of treating tuberculosis at home was based on five basic principles: 1) living, and especially sleeping, outdoors as much as possible; 2) absolute bedrest, on cots or reclining chairs; 3) drinking large quantities of milk and olive-oil; and 4) keeping daily records of body-temperature, weight and number of hours outdoors. The fifth essential element was the weekly group-meeting of fifteen or twenty patients, with a doctor and social worker or nurse, where reports of weight-gain were discussed and posted on the blackboard. Outdoor living was encouraged with an almost religious zeal. Patients were urged to sleep on every kind of porch or verandah, in backyards and on tenement rooftops, and on special balconies built for the purpose. Army wall-tents, 7 x 7 feet with an extra fly, were recommended for rain and snow, with the sides rolled up whenever possible, winter and summer. If no outdoor sleeping-place could be arranged, special church funds were raised to move entire families to suitable facilities.

Pratt emphasized "isolating the source of the infection," namely the sick patient, by reducing the visits of family and friends. The weekly group-meetings, however, were a required feature of treatment, "held in a large cheerful room" at the hospital. They included "a pleasant social hour," bringing together patients of "widely different races and different sects [who] have a common bond in a common disease." The group discussions contained instructions on how to maintain their drastic regimen, vigorous encouragement about overcoming its problems, and lively reports of improvement. Records of greatest weight-gain and longest periods outdoors were posted, which "stimulated a spirit of healthy emulation. One patient was out-of-doors 706 hours in a month, an average of nearly 23 out of 24 . . . They never discuss their symptoms, and are almost invariably in good spirits.[12]"

During the early years of the tuberculosis classes there was no explicit acknowledgment of psychological factors, except to suggest that the groups should never be larger than twenty-five, and that "the doctor and friendly visitor must establish close personal relations with each member." But the importance of the group-meetings was obvious, as a powerful force in maintaining collective morale by a mutual identification through a common disease. The difficulties of adhering to such punishing physical conditions were also obvious, and the clinical results were correspondingly impressive. The statistics compared favorably with the best sanitaria of that period, and included many advanced cases that would have been refused admission at Rutland as untreatable.

After the first two years of the class method, Pratt reported that twenty-nine patients had "graduated" and returned to work, nine had died, five had been "discharged for disobedience" (that is, failing to follow the regime), and twenty remained in the group. In a later report,[13] Pratt defended the term "class," despite its authoritarian sound, because it implied some form of instruction. He also described the application of the class method to other conditions, by Richard C. Cabot at the Massachusetts General Hospital, by W. R. P. Emerson with undernourished children, with diabetics by W. G. Smillie, and with obese patients by a Mrs. Jacobson, a social worker at the Peter Bent Brigham Hospital.

Pratt was asked why so many tuberculosis classes that started elsewhere had not survived, while the Emmanuel Church class and "its daughter," the Arlington Street Church class, had continued successfully for fifteen years. Pratt suggested two elements: the importance of "a professional and not a volunteer social worker," and the influence of the therapists' personalities. The Christ Church class in New York, for example, had obtained remarkable results for four years, until the social worker married "and the class soon ceased to exist." In a discussion about the doctor's personality, Pratt stressed the greater importance of the social worker, compared to the doctor: "it would be more correct to say that it is the woman who is everything."

Several decades later, Pratt[14] described his results in treating neuroses and functional disorders at Boston Dispensary, from 1930 to 1952. By that time he called his class method "group psychotherapy," but he began by recalling his first interest in treating nervous conditions in 1913, when he met Isador Coriat on the steps of the Boston Medical Library. Coriat had a copy of Déjérine's book, just translated by Smith Ely Jelliffe,[15] which he enthusiastically recommended to Pratt. Déjérine's emphasis on "emotional *re-education* and persuasion" (italics added) appealed to Pratt, and he quoted

> Psychotherapy depends wholly and exclusively upon the beneficial influence of one person on another. One does not cure an hysteric or a neurasthenic . . . by reasoning or syllogisms. They are only cured when they come to believe in you.[16]

Pratt referred to similar sentiments, about treating the patient, not the disease, expressed by various physicians. He mentioned Francis Peabody and Rudolph Krehl, both mentors of his, and quoted from James Jackson's 1855 *Letters to a Young Physician*.[17] "The priest had the parish for his cure, the physician the sick for his."

More explicitly than Edes or Cabot, Pratt believed that all physicians should be able to treat "the common neuroses," and that these conditions were best treated by general physicians, not by psychiatrists. Referring to a colleague who believed all neurotic patients should be referred to the psychiatry clinic, Pratt wrote "He should have known better. The treatment of the simple neuroses belongs in the field of general medicine . . . I might add that the psychiatrist is often confused as to the significance of bodily symptoms," as in ordering lab-procedures the internist would know were unnecessary. Nevertheless, he personally admired and collaborated with a number of psychiatrists, including Merrill Moore and Herbert Harris. And in spite of his doubts about psychiatrists' lack of skill in physical diagnosis, he encouraged non-physicians, namely ministers and divinity students, to practice group psychotherapy "under medical supervision."

In his 1953 paper, Pratt reviewed the results of twenty-two years of the class method at the Dispensary. He estimated that thirty-six percent of all medical patients were suffering from nervous disorders, whatever their physical symptoms might be. Cabot in 1908 had suggested "two fifths, probably more nearly one half." Pratt reported that

3,434 patients had been referred to group psychotherapy, eighty-four percent had attended more than one meeting, and fifty-six percent had attended five or more times. He wrote "A large percentage report that they are much improved. Many state that their symptoms have entirely disappeared. To our astonishment a large number continue to attend the meetings after their recovery." He gave the example of a woman who had attended 619 meetings, although her "severe manifestations of hysteria, mistaken for chronic arthritis," had cleared up within the first few weeks.

As Pratt described the group-meetings, he began each session with an informal talk, "appealing primarily to the emotions of the members; I did not reason by argument, which, as Déjérine has pointed out, is not sufficient in itself to change the state of mind." Although these were patients with nervous disorders, with whom little instruction was called for, some school-room features of the old tuberculosis classes persisted. There was a roll-call: each patient gave his or her name and the number of sessions attended. Slips were passed out, on which each patient described his present condition; these were collected and arranged in three piles: "feeling well," "a little better," and unchanged. Reports were read aloud, followed by questions, discussion and "a brief relaxation exercise with eyes closed." Appointments for individual interviews with a psychiatrist or psychologist were made for patients from the "unimproved" pile of slips. There was no separate pile for "feeling worse."

In an earlier paper, Pratt[18] had given a fuller account of his initial individual interview, in which he encouraged each patient to talk about their entire lives. He tried to point out connections between their physical complaints and underlying emotional conflicts, but he admitted that Déjérine's "moral re-education" was, in fact, "a form of faith cure." Pratt regarded his relaxation exercises as "really a mild hypnotic suggestion," following the technique of Prof. Elton Mayo. The school-room atmosphere persisted in the seating-arrangements, according to each patient's attendance-record, with "the four [patients] with the highest score" on a settee beside the class leader. This arrangement was proposed by Dr. George Gehring during a visit to a class, so "the newcomers could see what he termed the radiance of their faces."

The size of Pratt's groups remained about fifteen to twenty, as in his original tuberculosis classes, which he never referred to, strangely enough, in his papers on the group treatment of neuroses. In his 1946 paper Pratt explained the origin of his term "Thought-Control Clinic," from the words of a patient, who explained to a neighbor that her cure was "not a miracle, from visiting Father Power's grave [but] from Dr. Pratt's thought control class." Pratt approved of his patient's formulation and adopted her name, "thought-control," for his method because "that cure was wrought by thought and emotional control. A strong vitalizing emotion had removed her pain, but the underlying cause had been eradicated by an altered state of mind; in other words by moral re-education as Déjérine termed it."

These homely details reflect the basic elements that Pratt adhered to throughout his long career as a group-therapist, from 1905 to 1953. These elements may seem naïve in retrospect, with their echoes of the classroom and Sunday school, but the effectiveness of a group-identification through a shared disease is recognizable in many group methods, like Alcoholics Anonymous and other self-help groups. In the original tuberculosis classes, a quasi-religious belief in the virtues of outdoor living had a unifying effect, enhanced by the sharing of its rigors. The attention paid to maintaining good attendance itself may have had a similar effect in the later Thought-Control Classes. Pratt acknowledged these elements, and the fact that his patients' submission to a group leader followed Oslerian precepts of obedience to medical authority.

Pratt accepted his belated recognition as a founding-father of the group-psychotherapy movement at a celebration for his sixtieth birthday, when he was given a thousand-page *Festschrift* of writings by his admirers. In 1955, a year before his death, another meeting was held in his honor, called *Fifty Years in Group Psychotherapy*,[19] for the occasion, six of Pratt's papers and selected essays on his method were reprinted.

The authoritarian elements in his method, and the charismatic effect of his own personality, were not unrecognized by Pratt's admirers. Cabot[20] wrote enthusiastically

> no class was as successful as his because there was only one Joe Pratt . . . No one was as warm-hearted as he, no one else enjoyed meeting his patients as much, was as pleased with every little success and as confident of eventual recovery. Hopefulness and buoyancy like his . . . make him a very powerful therapeutic instrument. [His patients] got well not wholly because they wanted to get well but largely because he wanted them to—a very queer and very human state of things.

Worcester gave a similar picture of his personality, as "kind, merry, highly skillful and optimistic," and summed up its effects succinctly: "Dr. Pratt was like a father surrounded by his children."[21]

In a review-article on various types of group-psychotherapy, Thomas[22] defined Pratt's method as "repressive-inspirational," according to a classification proposed by Merrill Moore. Harris,[23] who had worked with Pratt at the Boston Dispensary, quoted McDougall in explaining Pratt's clinical results: "group [behavior] is characterized by a submissive tendency on the part of the majority, separate from the gregarious tendency, and the operation of this instinct for submission constitutes the main cognitive power behind the suggestibility of the group." One of the foremost figures in the later development of group-therapy, S. R. Slavson,[24] wrote a thoughtful and sympathetic account of Pratt as a pioneer. Slavson suggested that Pratt, although he denied the influence of his own personality, somehow perceived "the acceptance [of] the therapist as a parent figure . . . which later came to be known as transference [before] the spread of Freud's formulations."

Although Pratt clearly enjoyed his belated recognition among group-therapists, a charming letter to George Shattuck[25] indicated that he had not forgotten his early rebuffs at the Massachusetts General Hospital:

> Your remark that in the early days of my career my elders mistook my enthusiasm for immaturity or worse is doubtless true. It set me thinking of the past. Years after Dr. Councilman, my father in medicine, had retired, I asked "why was I not advanced at the Harvard Medical School?" "That is an easy question to answer," he said, 'they didn't like you!"

Pratt also recalled a fellow-worker in the chemistry lab at Massachusetts General Hospital who asked him, "How is it you can be so cheerful, when you know that everyone around here hates you?" These disarmingly frank afterthoughts, about Pratt's rejection by Harvard and his search for a secure position at Tufts Medical School and the Boston Dispensary, reflect his innate optimism in response to adversity. This quality probably contributed to his sympathetic identification with his patients, whom he perceived in their adversity as underdogs and outcasts, and to his patients' unconscious identification with him.

5

The Beginnings of the Emmanuel Movement (1906–1909)

As we have seen, the local traditions of medical psychotherapy, and Joseph Pratt's creation of his "class method" for the treatment of tuberculosis, formed the elements from which the Emmanuel Movement evolved. Pratt's collaboration with Worcester began in 1905, when Pratt turned to Worcester for help. They worked closely together and made use of the Emmanuel Church for their group-meetings. Worcester's memoirs[1] recount the same dramatic beginnings and the first gratifying results that Pratt had reported, but Worcester disagreed with Pratt about what caused their patients' clinical improvement. Pratt attributed their results to bed-rest and fresh air, while Worcester "ascribed our remarkable success chiefly to Dr. Pratt's personality and to the faith and hope he was able to instill into our patients."

Worcester continued his collaboration with the tuberculosis classes for the next eighteen years, with meetings at the Church and expenses supported by church funds. At that time the Commonwealth of Massachusetts offered to take over the Emmanuel program for tuberculosis, and to continue its class method, boasting that even better results could be achieved. Worcester was skeptical and his doubts were confirmed when the state-supported classes dwindled and the program was given up after a few years. In eighteen years, Worcester wrote, boasting a little himself, "we cured more consumptives than Christian Science has cured in its entire history."

Worcester's initial contact with Pratt seemed to be a mutually beneficial coincidence, when Worcester had just arrived in Boston and was looking for an interesting social project. Pratt, in turn, needed both financial and logistical help in his experiment with the home-care treatment of tuberculosis. The encounter was influential in strengthening Worcester's strong medical orientation, when he applied Pratt's "class method" to the treatment of nervous disorders. Apparently Worcester sought no advice from his fellow clinical psychologists at Harvard, like William James, Hugo Münsterberg and Josiah Royce. His contact with James, whom he much admired, concerned a philosophic question about their old Leipzig professor Fechner, not the practice of psychotherapy that James had been so enthusiastic about. But Worcester soon found an ideal collaborator in a fellow clergyman, a Dr. Samuel McComb, who proved to have a background similar to his own. McComb was a witty, talkative, Anglicized Irishman who had studied psychology at Oxford. He had been influenced by Sir William Graham, a neurologist who was interested in psychotherapy, playing a part similar to Weir Mitchell's in Worcester's life.

Worcester later attributed one element of the Emmanuel Movement, the collaboration between clergy and medicine, to a jocular remark of Mitchell's,[2] that by working together "on the basis of sound religion and sound science" they could put a colleague they disliked "out of business." Other elements included Worcester's early interest in medical problems, and the vestiges of a healing tradition that he discovered in early Christianity, reflected in the bishop's consecration oath, "O Bishop heal the sick." He believed that modern psychology should be taught to both young clergymen and young doctors, when seminaries and medical schools were equally lacking in psychological education.

Between 1905 and 1906, with Dr. McComb as his associate, Worcester wrote[3] that he had consulted

> the most eminent physicians, surgeons and psychiatrists of Boston, New York and Baltimore and informed them that *if it met with their approval* we were thinking of forming a class, which we innocently supposed would be no larger than the Tuberculosis Class, for the moral and psychological treatment of nervous and psychic disorders. We carefully explained that we had no wish nor intention to intrude ourselves into the physicians' functions, for which we had no qualifications, but to place ourselves at their disposal and, in every way, to cooperate with them.

Had this approval been withheld, Worcester insisted, he and McComb would never have continued their efforts, because medical recognition was an essential feature of their method, one that distinguished "our undertaking from all healing cults whatsoever."

Following these consultations, the first meetings were to be held in November 1906, to begin with four "addresses" on successive Sunday evenings in the parish-house, "to audiences of moderate size." The first was given by James Jackson Putnam, then nearly sixty and probably the most respected neurologist in Boston. He was a leader of the psychotherapy movement, as we have seen. He was already experimenting with Freud's "cathartic method" at Massachusetts General Hospital, although he had not yet become a committed psychoanalyst. The second lecture was delivered by Richard Cabot, twenty years younger than Putnam, with whom he had collaborated in establishing social work at the Massachusetts General. The third and fourth lectures were given by Worcester and McComb, respectively, and they concluded with an announcement: they would be at the parish-house the next morning, along with two psychiatrists, "to meet with persons who might wish to consult us in regard to moral problems or psychical disorders."

On Monday morning, to their amazement, 198 men and women arrived, "suffering from some of the worst diseases known to man, old chronic maladies, rheumatism, paralysis, indigestion, conditions which lay wholly outside our province. Thus, from the very beginning, our carefully prepared scheme was taken out of our hands and committed to the people."[4] Their two psychiatrists, probably Putnam and Isador Coriat, their long-term collaborator, were dismayed by the crowd, to which a local asylum had contributed "several hack-loads of its patients to . . . have a joke on Dr. Putnam." Nevertheless the two physicians set about examining the patients and separating the organic from the functional, while the two clergymen interviewed them individually. Then the gathering sang a few hymns, and we "gave them something to eat and invited them to come again. Out of this ghastly group," Worcester concluded, "I formed our Health Conference for prayer and instruction" that was to meet weekly for nearly twenty years.

"We could have handled the situation we had created easily enough if it had not been for the newspapers," Worcester later recalled,[5] but the press gave their meetings "undue prominence" and found them "an unending source of weird stories and caricature." The "better papers," meaning *The Boston Evening Transcript*, were reasonable, but "the sensational press seemed determined to find something wild and fanatical in our work . . . and when they could not they would invent it." These inventions included a story that in Philadelphia Worcester had raised a woman from the dead and was planning to repeat this feat in Boston. Thus newspaper publicity was a problem from the beginning, and had even created the name the "Emmanuel Movement." Worcester had initially deplored this name, just as Ernest Jones had objected to psychoanalysis being called a "movement," but the name was accepted for convenience's sake.

Inevitably this widespread publicity, both responsible and sensation-seeking, intensified the attacks from all quarters upon the Emmanuel Movement. Worcester recognized the effect on his congregation, "that reading lurid accounts of our doings . . . must have been a sore trial to them." He acknowledged the upper-class status of most of his parishioners, "refined, socially respectable, in fact élite," whose church was placed in the service of strangers, "a multitude of men and women, of all churches and of no church at all, which represented a cross-section of American society." If he had foreseen the ensuing "notoriety," Worcester wrote in 1932,[6] he would have consulted his vestry and congregation beforehand, and if they had objected he would have given up his undertaking. In that case, he speculated, the group meetings could have been moved elsewhere, and "we should have had no trouble in gathering another large congregation." But if they had left the Episcopal Church, Worcester and his allies would only have succeeded in "forming another despicable and short-lived sect (a thing abhorrent to me) . . . and forfeit[ing] the esteem of some of our best friends." In fact, Worcester concluded, his congregation and his bishop, at Trinity Cathedral, only a few blocks away, had proved to be remarkably tolerant about the "movement" that bore the name of their church.

In seeking a clear picture of what took place at the

weekly meetings themselves, the present-day reader will be amazed at the five enormous scrapbooks[7] that Worcester compiled between 1908 and 1916, with their closely-packed newspaper clippings from all parts of the United States and Great Britain. Instead of the fiery preaching and revivalistic atmosphere of mass-catharsis that the newspapers and magazines would lead one to expect, there was a bland and decorous mixture of academic psychology and informal group-discussion. The evening began in the parish hall with the singing of a few hymns, and there was a lecture by either Worcester or McComb and a physician or psychiatrist, on various topics in medicine or "psychopathology." A period for questions and informal discussion followed, with reports on individual problems, and the evening concluded with another hymn and light refreshments in an adjoining room.

Although Worcester had modeled his group on Pratt's tuberculosis class, the discussion was informal and open, without Pratt's emphasis on seating, roll-call and "obedience." There was no strict regimen to be followed, and the group was unified by sharing the experience of having a self-diagnosed nervous condition. Religion and medicine were represented by the hymns and the medical lecture, respectively, and the discussion centered around each patient's nervous symptoms. Thus Worcester's group-meetings in 1906 represent the first use of group psychotherapy, some twenty years before Pratt applied his "class method" to the treatment of neuroses at the Boston Dispensary. The popularity of the Emmanuel Movement was the result of many factors, including the dearth of other treatment resources, access to concomitant individual psychotherapy by Worcester, McComb and their medical colleagues, and the fact that treatment was free.

Among Worcester's medical associates, Putnam withdrew after his initial lecture, and Worcester's continuing supporters were Cabot, Pratt and Isador Coriat. Coriat was a young physician trained in both neurology under Morton Prince and in psychiatry at Worcester State Hospital. His interesting career[8] spanned the transition from the custodial care of psychoses to the suggestive psychotherapies and finally to psychoanalysis. Coriat later became Boston's second analyst in 1911, following Putnam, and still later was the founder of the second Boston Psychoanalytic Society in 1930.

Besides collaborating with Worcester and McComb in lecturing and treating individual patients at the Emmanuel Church, Coriat was a co-author of their book, *Religion and Medicine: The Moral Control of Mental Disorders.*[9] Like the Emmanuel Church meetings, this book proved unexpectedly popular, and went through three printings between May and November, 1908. Despite its title and connection with a church, only three of its twenty chapters dealt with religion; the rest, divided equally among the three authors, were almost indistinguishable in style. This is because all three authors were writing as "modern" psychologists, giving a readable, mildly didactic account of current "psychopathology" according to the French school. The discovery of "the subconscious mind" was hailed as "the most important advance which psychology has made since the days of Fechner and Weber." The general acceptance of this concept was attributed to William James, who showed that "the subconscious powers of the mind really exist." These powers were described in optimistic Jamesian terms as "reserve energies," to be released through psychotherapy for the benefit of man. The chapter on "Diseases of the Subconscious" was written by Coriat, as well as a chapter on treatment by means of suggestion. All the current authorities were referred to, from Schopenhauer and Edouard von Hartmann to Charcot, Janet and their American followers.

Examples of unconscious activity were drawn from hypnosis, conversion hysteria and multiple personality, and Coriat, who read German, already referred to Freud's *Neurosenlehre* and *The Psychopathology of Everyday Life*. About the latter, Coriat wrote rather casually: "In an interesting little volume, Freud has shown how great an influence is exerted by the subconscious on our everyday life. According to him, all dreams originate in our subconscious."[10] In a later book, Coriat[11] gave a fuller account of Freudian theory, referring to Freud's work on dreams, his Clark lectures and Putnam's paper about Freud. In the revised 1914 edition, after Coriat had become an analyst, he added a chapter on dreams and a clear account of the sexual etiology of hysteria. Except for his early references to Freud, Coriat's chapters were quite typical of contemporary writing on "psychopathology," from Weir Mitchell's neurasthenia to Janet's "psychasthenia" (a severe form of compulsion-neurosis.) *The Psychic Treatment of Nervous Disorders*,[12] by the Swiss, Paul Dubois, was mentioned as an important book, for its emphasis on persuasion and "moral re-education," just as Pratt had referred to Déjérine.

In Coriat's later book on abnormal psychology,[13] there was no popular appeal to the reader for using the book as a form of self-treatment, and the importance of medical evaluation and correct diagnosis was repeatedly stressed. Dramatic examples were given of errors in diagnosis: gastric cancer missed by being treated as neurasthenia, and hysterical symptoms intensified by unnecessary diagnostic procedures. Surprisingly, there was no reference in the book to the Emmanuel Movement or to the "class method" as a form of treatment. In fact there was little to differentiate *Religion and Medicine* from numerous other popular books by well-known psychologists like Boris Sidis,[14] Joseph Jastrow[15] and Hugo Münsterberg.[16]

The seemingly insatiable demand for these remarkably similar books is more significant than their actual contents.

Their popularity reflected a widespread yearning for information about emotional problems. Their very prose-styles and optimistic attitudes toward "cures" mirrored the temper of their times, the confluent movements for social and political improvement, for cultural modernism, that Hofstadter[17] called "The Age of Reform." The shift from the rural Mugwumps and Populists of the 1880s to the urban Progressives and radicals brought new audiences that were eager to read about "psychotherapeutics." The same men and women attended the innumerable lectures that Bostonians were teased about, and enrolled in various self-improvement classes. Earlier waves of enthusiasm for religious enlightenment were succeeded by fascination with social and scientific issues, from health fads to serious scientific and political controversies, from phrenology and spiritualism to Darwinism and Marxian theory, women's rights and the settlement house movement. As James had pointed out, the various "mind-cure" movements were welcomed for their optimistic environmentalism, in contrast to traditional European theories about heredity and mental illness as organic "degeneration" of the brain. This paralleled radical political theories that promised the cure of social ills by changing the society that had caused them. In a similar way French radicals in the late eighteenth century had once hailed Mesmerism for its promise of social betterment.[18]

Meanwhile changes in journalism and its readership had created a new audience for controversy about these social and cultural issues. Between 1870 and 1900, the circulation of daily newspapers had increased, from 2.8 to 24.2 million readers. New editors, besides the traditional reporting of events, "found themselves undertaking the more ambitious task of creating a mental world for the uprooted farmers and villagers who were coming to live in the city."[19] Most present-day journalistic techniques had been developed by the turn of the century: the personal interview, the special correspondents with their impressionistic accounts and subjective interpretations of the news. There were "feature articles" in the form of extended essays, and the active promotion of noble "causes," as well as stories about sensational stunts. Above all there was the "human interest story," for the poor to read about the follies and depravities of the rich, and for the rich and middle-class to read about the miseries of the poor. New popular magazines, like *McClure's* and *The Ladies' Home Journal*, reached audiences of 400,000 to a million, compared to the genteel old magazines like the *Atlantic* and *Harper's* that had circulations around 130,000. Whether the new journalism provoked or merely recorded the behavior of scientists and intellectuals, the press reported some significant differences between Europe and the United States.

If many American leaders of the new psychology wrote popular books about the topic, even more turned to public lectures and articles in the popular magazines, in addition to their traditional papers in scientific journals. A lively account of Prince's famous patient with multiple personality, Sally Beauchamp, appeared in *The Ladies' Home Companion* in 1908, and Putnam published an article on "The Nervous Breakdown" in the 1909 *Good Housekeeping*. Thus Worcester, in writing on the Emmanuel Movement for *The Ladies' Home Journal*, was merely following the practice of his colleagues in psychology and medicine. This was not the custom in Europe, where scientists usually published only in their own professional journals. Freud had deplored American habits of "popularization" even before he had experienced its effects, and his lectures at Clark University marked his only venture in addressing a popular audience.

In addition to *Religion and Medicine*, Worcester wrote and edited a series of pamphlets[20] which resembled further chapters from the book, and illustrated some cross-cultural currents of that era. Other authors included "Some End-Results of Surgery," by J. G. Mumford, a surgeon at the Massachusetts General Hospital, who warned against the dangers of sham-operations in the treatment of neurotic symptoms. Mumford also wrote on post-operative invalidism, fears of anesthesia and the value of visiting nurses during convalescence. A pamphlet by William James, *The Energies of Men,* was part of the series, a reprint from the *American Magazine* of his essay that became a popular book.[21] A future pamphlet by Josiah Royce was announced, to be called "Some Social Aspects of Mental Therapeutics," but this essay was never published. Sometime after 1908, a second book, planned as a sequel to *Religion and Medicine,* was withdrawn, by Worcester himself. This was "at some cost to ourselves," he wrote, because it was already set in type. His purpose was to avoid more publicity, and to spare the Emmanuel Movement further notoriety "by keeping silence and refusing to enter any controversy."

Besides the Sunday evening discussion-groups, which were a distinctive feature of the Emmanuel Movement, individual psychotherapy was offered by Worcester and his collaborators during the week, with office-hours in the parish-house and rectory and appointments made by telephone. From 9:30 in the morning to 2:30 or 3:00 PM, Worcester wrote,[22]

a constant procession of men and women passed through my study . . . I tried to give myself to each of these persons as if I had nothing else to live for, to put them at their ease, to enter into their problems with understanding and sympathy, not to hurry them, and also not to allow them to waste my time. As soon as one departed another came.

The length of his interviews or the duration of treatment

was not specified, but he came to know some of his patients "through a number of years." Worcester had so many phone-calls outside of clinic hours that he considered moving his telephone to the dining-room table, but his wife refused to permit this.

He recalled his clinical experiences with great pleasure, greater than Phillips Brooks', he surmised, "because [Brooks] lacked scientific method and the confidence and directness which such authority bestows." He also recalled that "when we began our work, Freud's name was unknown and psychoanalysis was not mentioned in America, but I stumbled on several of its leading ideas through my experience with my patients. The mere recognition and recitation of the terrors of the mind in some mysterious way seemed to mitigate them." His patients' conflicts, he discovered, usually went back "in some form to our early childhood and . . . they sprang from some childish fixation, repression, conflict or from the sense of inferiority impressed upon a child when its first timid approaches to life and reality were checked and thwarted."

He wrote in somewhat veiled terms about the importance of scientifically correct sexual information for children. He paid tribute to Coriat for selecting suitable patients, making diagnoses and recommendations, and "re-examin[ing] our patients from time to time to judge of our progress and of the success of our work." Though Worcester considered "the psychoneuroses the natural and legitimate field of our endeavor," he admitted that "no parochial clergyman" could limit himself to functional disorders and might be able to give comfort to "sufferers from physical disease."

Case-histories were sketchy and anecdotal, but they conveyed Worcester's confidence in a mixture of psychological commonsense, religious faith and the kind of hypnotic suggestion that was being used by other psychotherapists at that time. One example illustrated a risky encounter with a probably psychotic patient. After talking all evening with a brilliant, severely depressed fellow-minister, this patient became restless, "walking up and down and seemed hardly aware of my presence." When gently pressed for his thoughts, the patient replied, "I'm thinking of taking that poker and beating you to death." Without changing his expression, Worcester said "Just put that thought out of your mind. Do you suppose that's what I get for sitting here and talking to you all evening?" Though Worcester talked his patient into going back to bed in his hotel, next day the patient tried to push Mrs. McComb, his associate's wife, off a pier. Eventually psychiatric hospitalization was required. Worcester described this as an example of "insanity, a vain, unmeaning word," but admitted that when a patient was "unable to cooperate with his physicians and teachers, confinement becomes necessary."

A successful result illustrated the cure of a conversion-symptom, a type of case that was often reported in contemporary journals and is rarely seen today. A bright young architect was working on a new tuberculosis sanitarium that was being built for Worcester's friend, Dr. Mumford. After a prolonged exposure to cold, the architect reached his car in a state of collapse. When he awoke the next morning his right arm was paralyzed in the sense that it was incapable of voluntary movement; his right knee was ankylosed, being drawn up so that it was near his chin, and in that position it was clamped so firmly that it could not be moved by any method his physicians dared try. At this time his wife, who may have had other reasons, left him, taking his only child.

By the time Worcester saw this man, Mumford had amputated two toes that had become gangrenous because of his bizarre position. The patient's mental state was "the spiritual condition of a mad dog. He blasphemed God for bringing such misfortunes on him, and cursed me roundly for daring to think I could help him."

In a first brief encounter, Worcester suggested that his future was determined by faith, not reason, and that even if God Himself spoke to the patient now, he would not hear Him. When the patient seemed more accessible on a second visit to his hospital room, Worcester proposed his "first lesson." After a short talk on God's unlimited forgiveness, Worcester explained his method of relaxation, and under soothing suggestions he sank into a deep sleep. "Then I impressed upon him the command to obey me. I proceeded somewhat as follows, 'George, I know that you are not really paralyzed. You are able to move your arm and I wish you to move it now.' Without apparent effort, he raised his arm above his head . . . and shook hands with me." After deepening the hypnotic trance, Worcester proposed that he move his leg. The patient protested that it would hurt, but Worcester said he would be very gentle and not hurt him at all. "And with very little effort I straightened it out and placed it beside the other leg on the *chaise longue* where it remained." Then he summoned Mumford and the nurse, and after a few days in which the patient resumed walking, Worcester pronounced him cured.

This kind of hypnotic cure, the instant removal of a major hysterical conversion-symptom under powerful sugges-tion, had been obtained by Charcot some thirty-five years before. Despite Worcester's knowledge of unconscious forces, he described no exploration of emotional factors in this case, such as why the architect might unconsciously have "needed" to create this symptom. But the cure of such a severe disability certainly impressed the patient's physi-cian, Dr. Mumford, and a small number of doctors and clergymen who were friendly to Worcester or had personal experience with his clinical work.

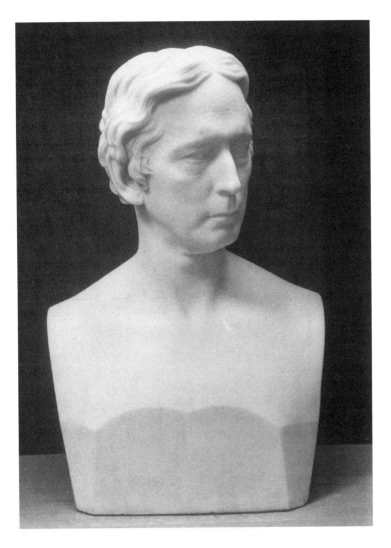

White marble bust by Horatio Greenough of Thomas Worcester, founder of the Swedenborgian Church of the New Jerusalem in Boston in 1818. Courtesy of the Church of the New Jerusalem, Beacon Hill, Boston. Photograph by Rick Stafford, Sackler Museum, Harvard University.

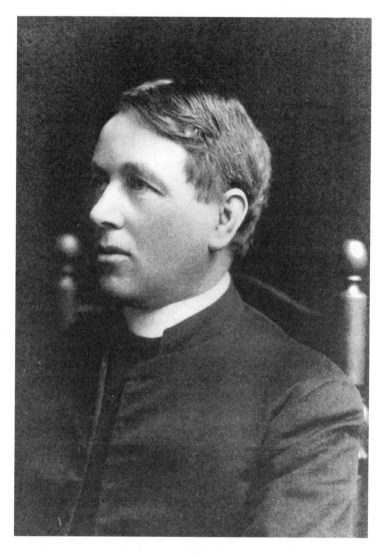

Photograph of Dr. Worcester taken shortly after his arrival in Boston in 1904. Courtesy of the Episcopal Diocesan Library, Boston.

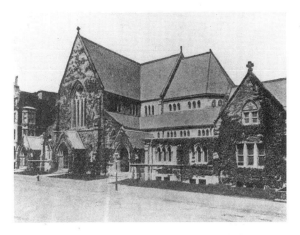

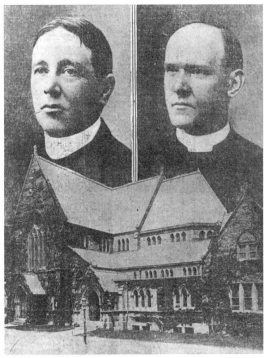

Above: The Emmanuel Church, Newbury Street, Boston, 1907; Below: Newspaper layout of "Leaders in Emmanuel Church Work," published in the *Boston Herald* on May 17, 1908. Elwood Worcester is depicted on the left and Samuel McComb on the right.

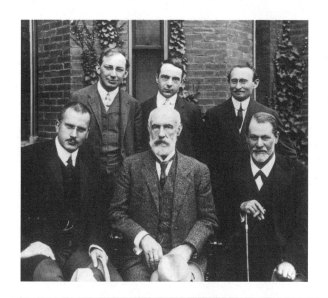

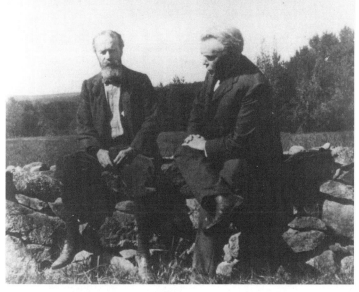

Above: Photograph taken at the Clark University lectures, September 1909. Back row, left to right, Sandor Ferenczi, Ernest Jones, A. A. Brill; front row, left to right, C. G. Jung, G. Stanley Hall, Sigmund Freud. Below: William James, left, and Josiah Royce, right, taken about 1908. Courtesy of the Francis A. Countway Library of Medicine, Boston.

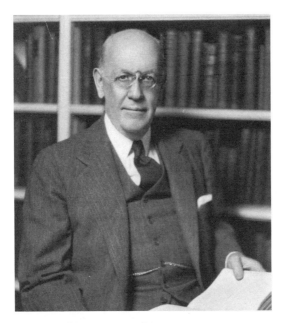

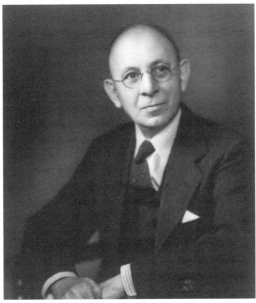

Above: Joseph Hersey Pratt (1872–1956) in later life; Below: Isador H. Coriat (1875–1943). Courtesy of The Countway Library of Medicine, Boston.

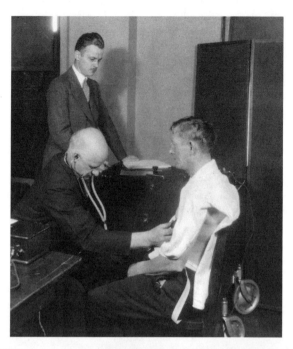

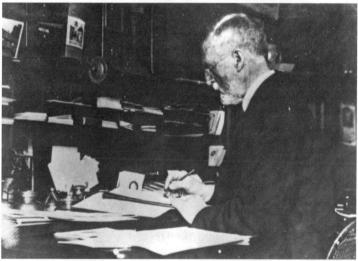

Above: Richard Clark Cabot (1868–1939) examining a patient ca. 1927; Below: James Jackson Putnam (1846–1918) in his study ca. 1910. Courtesy of The Francis A. Countway Library of Medicine, Boston.

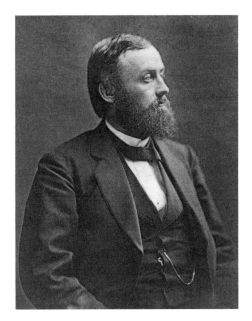

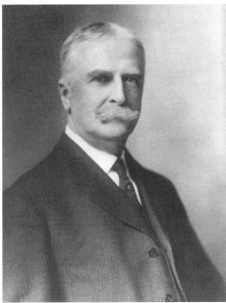

Above: Robert Thaxter Edes (1838–1923); Below: Frederick Henry Gerrish (1845–1920). Courtesy of The Francis A. Countway Library of Medicine, Boston.

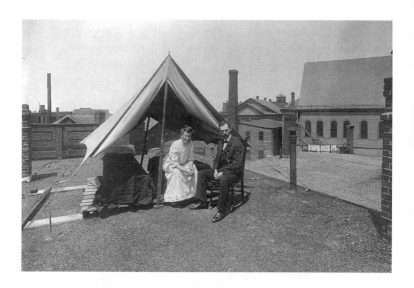

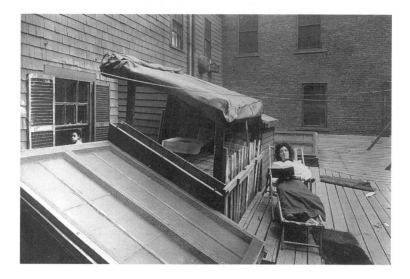

Photographs of Joseph H. Pratt's "fresh air treatment" of tuberculosis, Boston, 1912. Above: The husband and wife pictured here recovered their earning power by resting on this roof for about six months; Below, "Shack on roof used by patient living in a poor congested district of the city; she recovered completely without leaving her home and is now at work." Courtesy of The Francis A. Countway Library of Medicine, Boston.

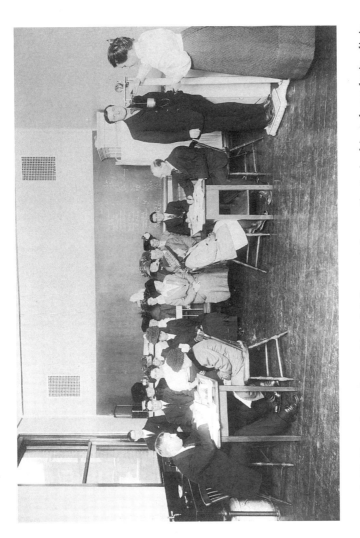

Joseph H. Pratt (seated at table, right) examining patients in his tuberculosis clinic ca. 1912. Courtesy of The Francis A. Countway Library of Medicine, Boston.

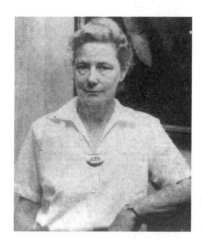
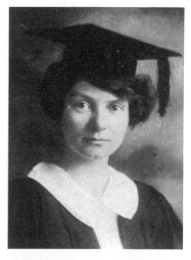
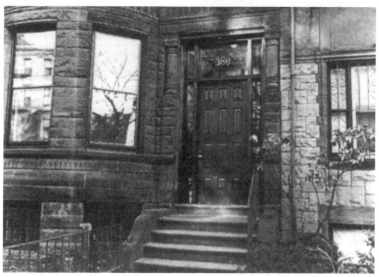

Above: left, Constance Worcester pictured during an interview by the *Boston Traveler*, July 22, 1954; right, Dr. Blandina Worcester (Mrs. Carroll Brewster), from her Radcliffe College yearbook, 1923; Below: Entrance to the former Emmanuel Church rectory, donated to Dr. Elwood Worcester upon his retirement in 1929, and inherited by his daughter Constance. Courtesy of the Radcliffe College Archives.

6

Growth and Expansion of the Emmanuel Movement (1906–1909)

From the dramatic first meetings of the "Episcopal Healing Class" in November 1906, there was a steady growth over the next two years. With the publication of *Religion and Medicine,* the year 1908 seemed the high tide of popular acclaim for the Emmanuel Movement. This is illustrated by the five scrapbooks[1] that spanned the years 1906 to 1916: the first three and a half volumes were devoted to the year 1908. The scrapbooks reflect the public response to the Emmanuel Movement, because they contained newspaper and magazine articles collected from all over the United States by an early professional clipping-service. This was Henry Romeike Inc. ("The First Established and Most Complete Newspaper Cutting Bureau in the World," London 1881, New York 1884). Pasted on both sides of large folio pages, 120 to a volume, with many reprints and pamphlets laid in, the clippings come from every city, large and small, in the United States.

There was a smaller number from London, Northern Ireland and Scotland, and a few from Germany.

Coriat's scrapbook[2] (1906–1953), which also used a professional clipping-service, covered a wider range of articles loosely related to mental phenomena, from newspaper stories about dramatic amnesias and loss of identity to scientific meetings like the American Therapeutic Society and the Clark University lectures. Worcester's scrapbook focused more narrowly on the Emmanuel Movement itself, and its tuberculosis program which proceeded *pari pasu* with the "functional disease" classes. There were also occasional articles about faith-healing by other means, Christian Science, and spiritualism (communication with the dead through a medium, table-rapping etc.). Worcester was quoted as a public figure, apart from the Emmanuel Movement, as opposed to the performing of Richard Strauss' *Salomé,* and as defending St. Gaudens' statue of Phillips Brooks in Trinity Church, Copley Square, as "far from sacrilegious."

By December 1906 there were two meetings a week at the Emmanuel Church, on Wednesdays and Fridays at 8, one with as many as 300 patients, and the other with 200. The title of the discussion-groups was "The Psychic Treatment of Nervous Diseases," and medical supervision was emphasized from the beginning. There were "four eminent neurologists" to examine each patient and make sure that only "functional disorders" were being treated at the Emmanuel Church. Organic diseases, like tuberculosis, were referred elsewhere, although the Church was also treating tuberculosis patients that were selected for Dr. Pratt's small "classes" of fifteen to twenty. Individual treatment by Worcester and McComb, in what was called a "moral clinic," was conducted during the day, usually mornings, while the afternoons were reserved for house-calls.

Cabot[3] wrote a thoughtful article in a popular magazine,

reviewing the clinical records of the Emmanuel Church for March–November 1907. Of 178 cases, which represented half of those actually seen, forty-seven were much improved, twenty-eight slightly improved, forty-eight not improved and fifty-five lost to follow-up. Cabot considered these good results, and was pleased that only two patients had turned to Christian Science or New Thought. "For all but the very well-to-do, the [treatment] resources available are woefully inadequate . . . the average physician fights shy of [neurotic patients]; they bore him, fatigue him and annoy him." There are, he concluded, "great possibilities for good, and rather limited possibilities for harm."

During the first two years, the press was filled with reports from fellow clergymen of all Protestant denominations, most of them enthusiastic about the Emmanuel program. At least half a dozen had started programs of their own, following Worcester's principles, of whom the best-known were the Rev. Loring Batten of St. Mark's Parish, New York, Bishop Samuel Fallows of Chicago, and the Rev. A. Lyman Powell of Northampton, Massachusetts. Except for Cabot's support and Coriat's loyalty as a member of Worcester's original staff, physicians had been relatively silent. The first medical criticism came early in 1908, from Dr. Charles K. Mills of Philadelphia, where Worcester had visited to preach in his former parish of St. Stephen's, acknowledging Weir Mitchell as one of the sources of the Emmanuel Movement. Mills refused to question Worcester's sincerity and accepted hypnosis as having medical uses, but he attacked "Worcesterism" as a criticism of medicine and asked how long its cures would last.

In March 1908, Putnam was in New York, giving a lecture on "The Nervous Breakdown" at the New York Academy of Medicine. When asked his views about the Emmanuel Movement, Putnam[4] "spoke with great diffidence, said it was hard to put his current views into words." In brief, he feared physicians working with ministers in psychotherapy "might rebel at taking second place." But he granted that great benefits had been accomplished by Worcester's methods. In Philadelphia Worcester's work was assaulted by Francis X. Dercum, the arch-enemy of the new psychotherapy and later of Freud. He denounced "pastors in medicine" and "hypnotists" of all kinds. Weir Mitchell, once a friend of Worcester, criticized "not psychotherapy but its abuses," while Dr. Charles Dana defended the Emmanuel Movement.

By the summer of 1908, the Emmanuel Movement "had taken root in England," according to Bishop Winnington-Ingraham. Worcester's book was favorably reviewed, as "a conscientious attempt to reconcile faith healing with orthodox medical treatment." But there were excesses by over enthusiastic followers: a "Psycho-Therapeutic Hospital" in London that used neither drugs nor surgery but believed in the curative powers of "rays that emanated from certain persons." A clergyman in Albany, New York, claimed that he had cured his four year old daughter of "naughtiness" by verbal suggestions while she was sleeping. These questionable practices by so-called followers increased with time, and Worcester was always concerned about untrained imitators who failed to keep close cooperation with doctors. But he repeatedly declined to create any kind of national "movement" that might have enforced greater uniformity of methods.

A "summer school" for theology students was given on psychotherapy at the Emmanuel Church, by Worcester, McComb and Coriat, and a similar course for Tufts medical students was announced for the fall term, to be taught by Morton Prince and the Rev. A. B. Shields. In 1908 and 1909 an unusual popular journal was published, called *Psychotherapy,* edited by W. B. Parker[5] with collateral reading and "editorial aids." The first issue opened with a "general introduction" by Cabot, called "The American Type of Psychotherapy," in which he claimed that American physicians had resisted a "scientific, rational mind-cure" movement because they associated it with Christian Science, New Thought and other forms of faith healing. "In Europe, on the other hand, where there has been no movement among the laity, where psychotherapy has been wholly in the hands of the physicians, its scientific and reasonable sides have been developed." Cabot referred favorably to Dubois' work over the years, and the collaboration between clergy and physicians in the Emmanuel Movement. He emphasized that "mental treatment—-I mean 'mental' to include 'moral' and 'physical'—-does not cure cancer" or any other organic disease. But Cabot estimated that "not less than two-fifths (probably more nearly one-half) of all the cases of illness which the ordinary general practitioner sees" represent "treatable functional disorders." He acknowledged the commonsense origins of psychotherapy in the traditional doctor-patient relationship, and regretted the lack of psychological teaching in medical schools. As a result, he suggested, social workers were better equipped than most physicians in handling the emotional problems of patients.

Other issues of *Psychotherapy* contained an address by Putnam, "The Philosophy of Psychotherapy," and an article by the Rev. Loring W. Batten on "Healing in the Old Testament." Surprisingly, an official statement appeared from the British "Society of Emmanuel," a group totally unrelated to the Boston Emmanuel Movement. Unlike the Emmanuel Movement, the British Society "maintains that the healing, not merely of nervous and functional [symptoms], but also of organic disease is within the scope of the Church's office." Cancer-cures were attributed to the laying on of hands, and although the British organization noted the difference between the two groups, the editor of *Psychotherapy* suggested that the British Society was "taken up under rational scientific guidance" by the Emmanuel Church in Boston. This misleading note increased the confusion derived from the similarity of names.

In the second and third volumes of *Psychotherapy* there were two articles by A. A. Brill, soon to found the New York Psychoanalytic Society in 1911. Both articles gave clear accounts of psychoanalytic methods, including free-association and dream-interpretation, and reviewed Freud's *Psychopathology of Everyday Life*. Next came a review-article by Cabot on the psychotherapy movement, describing the principal figures from Janet, Déjérine and Dubois to Münsterberg, Jastrow and the Emmanuel Movement. He placed the Emmanuel Movement in the "middle ground," between the "hard" scientific observations of the French neurologists and the "soft" writers of popular inspiration like Horatio Dresser and Ralph Waldo Trine. Cabot described Breuer and Freud's theories of hysteria as "contain[ing] a considerable body of interesting facts" but he found the importance attached to sexual trauma "startling and, to me, inconclusive." This juxtaposition of Freud and the preanalytic therapies of suggestion illustrated the transitional features of the period, when both co-existed and psychoanalysis was partly accepted as another form of psychotherapy.

During the summer of 1908, press-coverage of the Emmanuel Movement continued to be favorable, with more clergymen setting up healing-programs modeled on the Emmanuel Movement. But in November an unsigned editorial appeared in the *Boston Medical and Surgical Journal*,[6] probably written by the editor, E. W. Taylor, an eminent neurologist and a member of Putnam's department at the Massachusetts General Hospital. After acknowledging that "the cornerstone of the movement is cooperation between the medical profession and the church," the editorial claimed that Boston physicians as a whole have "never stood behind the movement and [are] increasingly less inclined to do so." The basic criticism that emerged from the polite verbiage was that psychotherapy was being carried out by non-physicians. Since the chief advances in "mental therapeutics" were the work of "psychologists and physicians," treatment should remain in medical hands. Treatment by the clergy, in fact, "retards the progress in the only direction in which normal psychotherapeutics can grow—through the medium of the medical profession."

Shortly before this, as if synchronized with Taylor's editorial, Putnam had written two letters to the Boston *Herald*,[7] in order to explain his support of the Emmanuel Movement. He wrote that he now considered the Emmanuel Movement "a mistake," despite his regard for the sincerity of its founders, because clergymen were assuming clinical responsibilities that physicians are given "only after years of study and training." Putnam acknowledged that he had "cooperated with Dr. Worcester at the outset," referred occasional patients to the Emmanuel Clinic, and had never questioned their therapeutic results. Now, however, he had withdrawn his support when he realized "what the outcome would be," namely that the movement was spreading and being taken up by clergymen who were not as well qualified as Dr. Worcester.

Coriat replied to Putnam's letter, reiterating his and Dr. Worcester's belief in "absolute medical control" and describing their precautions about accurate diagnosis and the referral to other physicians of any patient who was organically ill. But this point, strongly emphasized when the first Emmanuel meetings were held two years before, was invariably ignored by physicians, once the tide of criticism by the medical Establishment had turned.

Already in September 1908, Putnam[8] had written Worcester what must have been a very painful personal letter, first to thank Worcester for his book, *Religion and*

Medicine, and then to acknowledge his growing reservations about the expansion of the Emmanuel Movement. The letter is tortured and circumstantial, with professions of friendship and personal esteem for Worcester, followed by concern about clergymen usurping the physician's role. Putnam apologized about the "unjustifiable length" of its eighteen pages, and for the seeming contradiction between his initial support for the Emmanuel Movement and his present position. In a labored attempt to define the relative roles of doctor and minister, Putnam adumbrated his later essay in the *Harvard Theological Review*,[9] concluding "I do not think the *success* of the movement to be a warrant for its value." His closing passages are a vague appeal to Worcester for "establishing *a new institution,*" in which medicine, the church, social work and others would join in a spirit of mutual criticism and cooperation.

Critical attacks on the Emmanuel Movement appeared in other cities, as Joseph Collins, President of the American Neurological Association, denounced the "healing mission" of the Rev. Batten in St. Mark's Parish, New York. An editorial in the *Medical Record*,[10] the New York equivalent of the *Boston Medical and Surgical Journal,* inveighed against another New York minister for "taking up the practice of medicine as part of his clerical work." As long as the Emmanuel Movement was confined to Boston, the editorial continued, it could be dismissed "as a sort of neo-Eddyism, one more of the many queer fads with which the citizens of that town are wont to amuse themselves."

Criticism of the Emmanuel Movement reached a climax in December 1908, with a front-page article in the Sunday *Boston Globe*,[11] reporting interviews and lengthy statements from the medical élite of the city. Putnam wrote in more forceful terms, calling "the whole affair an injury to the progress of scientific medicine, especially to neurology." He deplored the sensationalism, "notoriety" and newspaper

publicity generated by the Movement, calling it "an epidemic" that must be controlled. Again the main point of his
criticism was the danger of treatment by "untrained men,"
and the "enormous number of mentally sick people . . .
getting their psychotherapeutics from the wrong well." The
only new question he raised was whether organic and functional conditions could be so easily distinguished, when
neurasthenia, for example, might prove to have an organic
basis. (Putnam was referring to Janet, in one of his 1906
Boston lectures, an ally whom Putnam would later reject,
when he became an analyst.)

Putnam's remarks were followed by criticisms of the
Emmanuel Movement by Prof. Münsterberg of the Harvard
Psychology Department, and by physicians from the many
hospitals and medical schools of the city: Philip C. Knapp
and George Waterman of the Massachusetts General Hospital, J. J. Thomas of Tufts, Frank C. Richardson of Boston
University and W. N. Bullard of Carney Hospital. Most of
the doctors' objections were to treatment by non-physicians,
while Münsterberg, acknowledging the sincerity of Worcester, feared the "spread" of his methods to ill-trained hands.
In later comments, E. E. Southard,[12] chief of the progressive
new Boston Psychopathic Hospital, approved of the Emmanuel tuberculosis classes but he objected to the subordi-
nate position of physicians in psychotherapy; he also
rejected the concept of a "subconscious." Prof. G. Stanley
Hall,[13] of Clark University, called the Emmanuel Movement
"great" but foresaw the risk of "fill[ing] the mind with
dangerous superstition." Other critics joined the throng,
even from England, where Sir Dyce Duckworth (London
Times 1/17/09) condemned the Emmanuel Movement for
emanating from Boston, "a perennial source of false doctrine . . . which produces and contains more unstable men
and women than any other city I know."

After many patient attempts to defend their work by

Worcester, McComb and Coriat, and a major essay by Cabot justifying the Emmanuel Movement, a new policy was declared[14] by a board of four eminent physicians: Joel Goldthwaite, Richard Cabot, Mumford and Pratt. They were quoted in the *Boston Medical and Surgical Journal:*[15] "Dr. Worcester realizes the wisdom of discontinuing any semblance of a clinic." No more medical examinations were to be conducted at the Church and his medical staff was abolished. All patients for treatment were to be referred by their own physicians, and those without physicians were asked to choose one from an accepted list. Dr. Worcester "does not intend to treat disease. He simply stands ready to assist in the moral and spiritual re-education of any person whom a physician asks him to see . . . The physician must be in control throughout."

Following these controversies about the Emmanuel Movement in the daily newspapers, Putnam published his long, reflective essay in the *Harvard Theological Review,*[16] re-examining the respective roles of psychologists, physicians, clergymen and social workers in treating "nervous invalidism." This essay is essentially an endless equivocation, of less interest for the history of the Emmanuel Movement than for an understanding of Putnam's intellectual development. Though published in the summer issue, Putnam must have written this essay soon after the public debates of mid-winter 1908–1909, when he had just met Ernest Jones at Morton Prince's house,[17] and just before he became Boston's first psychoanalyst.

Unlike his harsh letters to the newspapers, Putnam was cautious in criticizing the Emmanuel Movement, emphasizing its "cordial recognition of scientific and medical authority" but still questioning its policy of encouraging "clergymen at large to act as practicing physicians." He acknowledged their therapeutic successes and the valuable role of non-physicians in drawing public attention to the needs of neurotic patients, but he questioned community endorsement of "a new form of medical specialty, represented by persons without adequate training."

In a footnote, Putnam was perhaps the only medical critic of lay psychotherapy to acknowledge the role of clinical psychologists in the mind-cure movement. He had previously recognized that Worcester and McComb were, in fact, trained in clinical psychology, but he now admitted that others (unnamed) had: "long been known" to give mental patients "advice and treatment through 'suggestion' and in kindred ways." The unnamed were, of course, eminent figures like William James, Münsterberg and the philosopher Josiah Royce, some of whom, like James, were his personal friends. But, having undermined a clear anti-lay psychotherapy position by admitting that *some* psychologists were qualified, Putnam attempted to minimize their importance, by adding that their work was *"always on such a small scale* [italics added] that the question of a new medical specialty had never arisen."

Putnam's essay continued to vacillate between doubting that the success of the popular psychotherapy movements was "a rebuke to [physicians] for not having paid more attention to their patients' mental and spiritual needs," and admitting that physicians, "and even neurologists . . . have been backward in the study and treatment of nervous invalidism." He paid homage to the church for "the recognition of a sort of public service in which all professions may unite," including doctors, ministers, teachers and the patients themselves. About teachers, Putnam quoted Helen Keller, in a rhapsodic passage about "her spirit sweeping skyward on eagle wings." He concluded with his admiration for Phillips Brooks, Emerson, the Emmanuel Church, and Richard Cabot for his work with social workers.

In striving toward a broad alliance of professions engaged in the treatment of nervous disorders, Putnam re-

jected the old dichotomy between teachers, clergy and social workers treating mental problems and physicians treating the body. But in defining separate roles he re-introduced
other dichotomies, assigning "character and motives" to the
church and the "skilled employment of special means of
preventing disease" to medicine. In these conflicting and
ambiguous attitudes toward religion and medicine, the
reader senses some conflicts in Putnam himself, torn between his old devotion to the psychotherapies of suggestion, and his new interest in psychoanalysis. There was also
his abiding concern with ethical issues, reflected in his later
book, *Human Motives*,[18] expounding a neo-Hegelian philosophy that he tried unsuccessfully to persuade Freud and
Jones to incorporate into psychoanalytic theory.[19]

There are further indications of Putnam's inner conflicts
in an unpublished letter to his old friend Henry P. Walcott,[20]
written after the public controversy over the Emmanuel
Movement had subsided. He was explaining his original
support for Worcester's work to his colleague: from knowing how many patients came to Worcester "for advice about
their mental and social troubles," and from admiring the
"surprising usefulness" of Pratt and Worcester's tuberculosis classes. Before the first public meeting in the church,
Putnam wrote, "I pictured . . . an organization of small
beginnings and slow growth," and gave only one short
address "on very simple lines." He emphasized that this
was a regular meeting of the church society and "not one
of the 'meetings,'" presumably one of the regular group-
discussions called "Classes in Moral Healing." He berated
himself for not having "done more thinking in the first
place," and referred again to "much that I disapproved of,"
and to features of the Emmanuel Movement that were "as
distasteful to me as it could be (I refer especially to the
public Wednesday evening meetings, with which I have
had nothing whatever to do.)"

Reading between the partly scratched-out lines, Putnam was undoubtedly referring, with such fastidious revulsion, to the regular discussion-groups, which he had never attended, that followed the first meeting. He was reacting as if the innocuous hymn-singing, commonsense homilies and reports of individual "cures" that he later heard about represented a kind of revivalistic mass-hysteria, like "speaking in tongues." Putnam had already acknowledged his distaste for newspaper publicity and "sensationalism," and he later confessed[21] that his initial reaction to Freudian theory had been similar, that he "rashly attributed these qualities to eccentricity and perhaps notoriety-seeking." He may also have been repelled by open manifestations of religiosity, in contrast to the austerities of Unitarian worship.

A similar fastidious distaste for publicity may have been a major element in Freud's condemnation of the Emmanuel Movement, shortly after Putnam's. Freud's only visit to this country, in September 1909, happened to coincide with continuing popular controversies about the Emmanuel Movement and lay-psychotherapy. In the light of Freud's early battles against the medical élite of Vienna and his life-long defense of lay-analysis,[22] it is surprising that he aligned himself with the Boston medical establishment. On his arrival from New York in 1909, even before his lectures at Clark University, Freud talked very freely to a reporter, Adelbert Albrecht,[23] who was fluent in German and had read and admired Freud's works. In this typically American newspaper interview, Freud was asked his opinion of the Emmanuel Movement, as a topic of current interest. Despite his mistrust of publicity, Freud held forth at some length:

> This Emmanuel Movement, which, however, I have not had time to study carefully, will die down as have so many other movements. When I think that there are many physicians who have been studying modern meth-

ods of psychotherapy for decades, and who yet practice it only with the greatest caution, this undertaking of a few men without medical—or with very superficial medical—-training, seems to me at the very least of questionable good. I can easily understand that the combination of church and psychotherapy appeals to the public, for the public has always had a certain weakness for everything that savors of mysteries and the mysterious, and these it probably suspects behind psychotherapy, which in reality has nothing, absolutely nothing mysterious about it. What may appear so is perhaps its great age, for it is in no sense a modern method of healing. It is the oldest therapy that medicine uses.

Freud was quoted as referring to a book by Richard Löwenfeld[24] that traced psychotherapy back to prehistoric times when doctors always placed patients in an obedient state of "faithful expectation." This was still true, Freud continued, and "we doctors could not give it up if we wanted to because the other party to our methods of healing—-namely the patient—-has not the slightest intention of doing without it." Freud referred to Bernheim at Nancy as the beginnings of modern psychotherapy, and went on to describe how his own method of psychoanalysis differed. But he also acknowledged that "we all practice psychotherapy, often without even knowing or intending it." Freud concluded, in a conciliatory vein, that "there are many sorts and ways of psychotherapy. All are good, if they accomplish their object, that is, effect a cure."

Among Freud's objections to the Emmanuel Movement, antipathy to the clergy was probably not a major element, because some months before, Freud[25] had welcomed the Swiss pastor, the Rev. Oscar Pfister, as a fellow-analyst, and reviewed a paper of his on pastoral psychotherapy. More likely Freud's objections were based on his distrust of Americans in general, and in particular of their predilection for popularization, as in his fears about diluting the "pure gold of analysis" with the baser metals of psychotherapy.

Brief as Freud's contact with the Emmanuel Movement was, in an American visit that was packed with other events so important for the future development of psychoanalysis, Freud still remembered the Emmanuel Movement many years later. He replied to the Rev. John Greene, a clergyman who was writing a history of the Movement,[26] in an only partly-published letter[27] of some interest. In the crotchety, opinionated style of his later years, Freud re-affirmed his abiding distaste for religion and his life-long mistrust of America:

> Dear Sir:
> I am naturally very surprised at the high esteem for my person which you express in your writing, and in order to make it bearable, I am thinking of the many smears to which I have been subjected and still am. In any case your utterances are a splendid indication of the freedom of your thinking, unchanged by theology. I find it very interesting that you know my grand-nephew Frederick Wiener. The announced work about the Emmanuel Movement I shall read with care. Perhaps one should be sorry that so much energy in America has been poured forth in these religious movements. But America is over-rich in energy.
> With best wishes, Your Freud.

Freud's disdain for the United States as a land of religious movements recalls similar sentiments about Israel, a few years before in a letter to Arnold Zweig:[28] "Palestine has never produced anything but religions, sacred frenzies, presumptuous attempts to overcome the outer world of appearance by means of the inner world of wishful thinking."

Freud's prejudices against all things American are well-known, as in blaming his indigestion on American food during his 1909 sojourn. So is his antipathy to religion in any form, glorying in proclaiming himself a "godless Jew." And the Rev. Green's inquiry enabled him to express both attitudes with some wry humor. Ernest Jones, like most European intellectuals, would probably have shared Freud's amusement, while William James and James Jackson Putnam had more difficulty freeing themselves from their nineteenth century American religious background.

7

Reorganization and Decline, 1909–1929

The year of maximum expansion and fiercest controversy was 1909, when the Emmanuel Movement evoked a volatile mixture of favorable and highly critical opinions from the public. The British *Lancet*,[1] for example, reviewed Worcester's original book, *Religion and Medicine*, beginning with a scornful reference to Beard's "American nervousness." The review condemned

> the ensuing flood of literature professing to cure such diseases by other than medical means, while strange doctrines enunciated in wild and often uncouth language, sometimes associated with mystical tenets disguised in pseudo-metaphysical phraseology, have been preached by innumerable disciples of the various American sects of mental, moral and spiritual healing.

After this abusive anti-American broadside, however, the reviewer acknowledged that medicine had long recognized the influence of mind on body. He commended the book for its chapters on psychotherapy, and for their clear, readable presentation. His only real criticism was Worcester's acceptance of the theories of Janet, which were not as popular in England as in the United States.

An interesting rebuttal to medical critics of the Emmanuel Movement came from an American journalist, H. Addington Bruce, who noted the ironic fact that with some noteworthy exceptions, the medical men of this country have signally failed to profit by the discoveries of the psychopathologists, and through their attitude of contemptuous indifference are themselves largely responsible for the successful development of non-scientific systems of psychotherapy.[2]

Edes and Putnam had made the same complaint, about the deficiencies in medical education, some dozen years before. According to Bruce, the work of Prince, Sidis and others continued to be "studiously ignored" by most physicians. In his opinion the Emmanuel Movement served a valuable purpose, "to galvanize them into belated action," in establishing hospitals, clinics and professorships for psychotherapy. But Bruce was not uncritical of the Emmanuel Movement, "as a therapeutic system . . . fraught with grave possibilities of danger to the community."

From among the psychologists, who might have found common cause with Worcester as a colleague, Prof. Lightner Witmer of Philadelphia launched a massive three-part assault on the Emmanuel Movement, in his own journal.[3] Possessing a Ph.D. from Wundt's laboratory himself, Witmer questioned Worcester's right to represent himself as a follower of Wundt or of Fechner. He claimed that the psychology of the Emmanuel Movement was the psychology of Hudson, Bramwell and Myers, in other words the methods of hypnosis and suggestion.

Witmer reviewed the history of experimental psychology in Wundt's lab, from 1879 when he had studied there, to 1888 when he became professor at the University of Pennsylvania. He praised Pratt's original tuberculosis classes, as promising "important and necessary social work," but he concluded that Worcester had "addled a very good egg through a premature exploitation of his work." Witmer objected to the use of hypnosis by clergymen, and to hypnosis itself as a method of treatment. Witmer assailed both Worcester's and William James's concept of the unconscious, calling James "the spoiled child of American psychology, exempt from all serious criticism." He considered James dangerous because he "us[ed] his professional authority to build up a modern occultism." Witmer concluded his diatribe against James with a few jabs at Putnam, "as one more instance of the scientific 'slush' whose source is . . . James' example and teaching." He also attacked Royce, by association, for his obscurantism.

Of the three physicians who had been actively engaged with Worcester and McComb in establishing the Emmanuel Movement, Pratt, Cabot and Coriat, all remained loyal in spite of the onslaught from medical critics. Coriat, as a co-author of *Religion and Medicine* and a member of the team that examined patients at the church clinic, had often acted as an official spokesman and answered Putnam's criticisms in the press. Pratt never criticized Worcester, except for his puzzling late-life denial of any link between the Emmanuel Movement and his "thought-control classes" at the Boston Dispensary.[4] In 1916 Pratt[5] was still praising the Emmanuel Church for its financial support of his tuberculosis classes. All his patients cured in one year, he reported, earned $50,000, while the total cost of the Emmanuel Movement program was only $15,000 for a ten-year period.

In his preachy style, Cabot continued to write enthusiastically about the Emmanuel Movement, for "assisting a large body of sad, dispirited men and women to face the problems of life more cheerfully, in consoling the distressed, in guiding the doubtful, in counseling the despondent, and in deterring persons meditating suicide from the accomplishment of this purpose."[6] But in 1931 Cabot did confess to Greene that he had gradually withdrawn from the Emmanuel Movement in recent years, not because he doubted its clinical usefulness but because he was "regarded as a 'scab' by most of his colleagues, and [was] losing professional prestige and chances of promotion."

In September 1909, the Rev. Albert C. Shields of South Boston was invited to San Francisco, to head a psychotherapy service at St. Luke's Hospital, modeled on the Emmanuel Movement. The following year Shields resigned his post, explaining that he was unable to establish his treatment program, but he vigorously denied that this represented a failure for the Emmanuel Movement. Many cures were effected but other obstacles "proved the impracticability of a psychopathic ward in a general hospital, where the evidence of sickness and suffering, and other 'nameless horrors'. . . act as depressing suggestions upon sensitive nervous patients."

The reorganization of the Emmanuel Church program had taken place early in 1909, with new rules and a distinguished medical advisory board, "to bring the physician and minister in closer cooperation." The Wednesday evening group-meetings continued as before, but referrals for individual psychotherapy were accepted only from physicians. Usually this was the patient's family doctor or a neurologist like Putnam, who continued referring patients long after he had withdrawn from the Emmanuel Movement. Self-referred patients without their own doctors were asked to choose from a list of recognized physicians for a physical examination.

In spite of these efforts to re-affirm the principle that "an internist remains throughout in charge of every case," the Boston medical community was still not satisfied. J. J. Thomas admitted that the new rules were an improvement but failed to "go to the root of the matter: clergymen will still go on giving medical treatment." Another physician, J. W. Courtney, wrote that "the subject has been discussed so much that the profession as a whole does not care one way or the other. In fact, the whole discussion has become tiresome."

Among other public figures, William James, who had welcomed all forms of psychotherapy to the "mind-cure movement," praised Worcester's recent book about Fechner. In his Hibbert Lectures[7] of 1909, James had expressed his admiration for Fechner, but in the same year he had strongly disparaged him, while praising the Emmanuel Movement:[8]

> Fechner is indeed a dear, and I am so glad to have introduced, so to speak, his speculations to the English world, although the Rev. Worcester has done so in a somewhat more limited manner in a recent book called *The Living Word*. (Worcester of Emmanuel Church, I mean, whom everyone has now begun to fall afoul of, for trying to reanimate the Church's healing virtue.) Another case of newspaper crime! The reporters got hold of it with their megaphones, and made the nation sick of the sound of its name.

Later in the same year, James had written to Flournoy, the well-known Swiss neurologist, about his mixed reactions to Freud's lectures at Clark University. In this often misquoted letter,[9] James expressed both his hope that "Freud and his pupils will push their ideas to their utmost limits, so that we may learn what they are. They can't fail to throw light on human nature; but I confess that he made on me personally the impression of a man obsessed with fixed ideas." James also chided Freud for criticizing the Emmanuel Movement: "A newspaper report of the congress said that Freud had condemned the American religious therapy (which has such extensive results) as very 'dangerous' because so 'unscientific.' Bah!" Thus Freud and James had found themselves on opposite sides of this public controversy about religion and lay-psychotherapy, when Freud usually opposed religion and defended lay-psycho-analysis.[10]

After the winter of 1909–10, according to the number of clippings in both Coriat's and Worcester's scrapbooks, there was a rapid falling-off in public notices of the Emmanuel Movement. Perhaps a dozen articles appeared in 1910, many reporting successes in far-off places, from Los Angeles to Brixton, England. Even in China, a missionary hospital in Wu Shi was built on land donated by a grateful patient, cured by the methods of the Emmanuel Movement. There were respectful reviews of books by its leaders, *The Christian Religion as a Healing Power*[11] by Worcester and McComb, and Coriat's[12] *Abnormal Psychology.* Other public activities of Worcester were noted in the press: preaching a memorial service at Appleton Chapel, or defending St. Gaudens' unorthodox statue of Phillips Brooks. McComb's travels and lectures were reported, and in 1915 his departure for Baltimore, to become rector of his own church, was accepted with regrets and warm appreciations of his work.

In 1911, replying to an inquiry about the Emmanuel Movement, Worcester and McComb reported[13] that they "continue to receive callers every morning," in other words patients for psychotherapy. The annual statistics for the Emmanuel Church[14] listed 925 members, with an additional 546 in its South End "mission," the Church of the Ascension. In the following year, articles in popular magazines "ceased abruptly [and] little or no serious reference to the work was to be found," according to Greene.[15] He attributed this falling off partly to loss of novelty, but primarily to Worcester's decision "to reverse their policy of engaging in controversy."

Worcester's scrapbooks confirm this for newspaper coverage, with a brief article or two each year from 1912 to 1916. At that time a "Health Conference" was held at the Emmanuel Movement Church,[16] to discuss the question "Have the Years Brought Changes?" The speakers reported that ten years of weekly health conferences had been completed, meaning the Wednesday evening discussion-groups, with an average attendance of 150 at each meeting. Dr. Pratt's tuberculosis classes were continuing, but they were now held in a room at Massachusetts General Hospital instead of the Church rectory. The success of a new feature was announced, Mr. Courtenay Baylor's group-discussions for "men who wish to put a stop to the habits that are wrecking their lives."

These meetings for self-referred alcoholics had first been described in 1911, when they were conducted by Ernest Jacoby, a lay-member of the congregation who had been cured of alcoholism by Dr. Worcester. These group-meetings for alcoholics had continued, sometimes called the "Jacoby Club," meeting separately from the larger Wednesday evening Health Conferences, in a comfortable basement room in the church. In 1912, Courtenay Baylor took over these group-meetings, as another lay volunteer, listed as a "friendly visitor" in the church's Social Service Department. He was a successful businessman who had also been cured of alcoholism by Dr. Worcester. He gave up his insurance business and devoted himself full-time to the church clinic, apparently as the first paid lay-therapist in the treatment of alcoholism. He opened his group-meetings to include men with drug-dependence as well as alcoholism, and requested an initial attendance for at least five sessions. There was no mention of women with either alcohol or drug problems, and at some point the so-called "men's group" was moved outside the church, to a house at 176 Marlborough Street, near Worcester's house at Number 186.

The later years of the Emmanuel Movement were described in two of Worcester's own books, *Body, Mind and Spirit,* written with McComb as a sequel to *Religion and Medicine,* and his entertaining autobiography, *Life's Adventure.* From 1912 to Worcester's retirement as Rector in 1929, according to Greene, Worcester continued his work quietly and unobtrusively, with weekly group-meetings and individual psychotherapy. He kept to his consistent policy of "allowing his associates to work out their own ideas. Everyone naturally had his own peculiar method of mental contact, and this was not interrupted." These associates included Baylor, whom Greene described as treating patients "with a more worldly approach," compared to Dr. Worcester, because of his business experience.

Worcester's own case-histories indicated that therapeutic relationships of some intensity were sustained over considerable periods of time, and reflected some changes in technique over the years. All the familiar neurotic syndromes were treated, with a high proportion of hysterical conversion symptoms, hypochondria and neurasthenia. These are the conditions that would be expected in that era, among patients who were self-referred or sent by doctors who had found "no organic disease." They illustrated their referring physicians' continued use of placebos and sham operations, as in a woman with *globus hystericus.* Her surgeon had proposed "a slight operation on the esophagus," combined with strong assurances that her symptoms would never recur. Worcester dissuaded her surgeon from this procedure and cured the patient after a few sessions, in which he interpreted her symptoms on the basis of an obvious pregnancy-dream.

Besides the many alcoholics, character disorders were also treated, as well as homosexuals and some psychotic patients. In spite of Cabot's advice never to treat severely depressed or manic-depressive patients, Worcester believed that no one seeking help should be refused treatment. He was proud of the fact that no patient had committed suicide while they were in treatment at the church clinic, over a period of some thirty years. These substantial successes in suicide-prevention would be highly impressive in any era, with any method of treatment.

By 1931, when Worcester and McComb wrote their second book, McComb had long been settled in Baltimore, and Coriat, their other co-author in the early years of the Emmanuel Movement, had become Boston's leading psychoanalyst, the successor to James Jackson Putnam. Worcester and McComb acknowledged how much psychotherapy had changed over some twenty-five years, and that "the psychology and science [in their first book] was entirely out of date." Their style was unchanged: warm-hearted, humorous and crotchety, sometimes naive but with a charm that recalled Worcester's other writings. For a man of sixty-nine with his clerical background, Worcester was generous in his praise of Sigmund Freud and courageous in defending his more unpopular theories. He was also able to disagree strongly with Freudian ideas he could not accept.

As a self-styled eclectic, Worcester wrote "I do not feel worthy to count myself one of Freud's disciples except in a very limited sense." He repeatedly paid homage to Freud for "discovering a new key to the understanding of human nature," and especially for the recognition of childhood sexuality "as a truth of the highest value." He accepted the psychoanalytic theory of dreams for "its amazing capacity to discover law where all is chaos," and the importance of sexual symbolism in dream-interpretation. He was critical of the Oedipus complex, however, and shrewdly debated one of Brill's crude arguments in support of it. And, as might be expected from his therapeutic optimism, he was deeply disturbed by the "essential pessimism" of Freud's concept of the Unconscious. "Few more terrible passages," he wrote, "occur in literature than [Freud's] description of this monster's struggle for liberty . . . even St. Paul never exceeded this arraignment of human nature." Like Putnam, Worcester disliked Freud's "materialism," meaning both his scientific determinism and his rejection of religion. Though attracted by Jung's religious and mystical interests, as many other clergymen had been, Worcester rejected Jung's personality-types as confusing and clinically useless.

Some of Worcester's misunderstandings of Freud were personal and idiosyncratic, but others resulted from the state of psychoanalytic theory at that time. This was just before the arrival of the émigré analysts and the systematizing trends of ego-psychology in the late 1930s and '40s. The present-day reader will still be impressed by Worcester's responsiveness to Freudian theory, and his tact and sensitivity as a clinician, as in treating severely depressed patients and evaluating suicidal risk. Though Worcester valued free-association and dream-interpretation, he also understood when such uncovering techniques were inappropriate, as in acute grief-reactions.

8

Worcester in Retirement and Successors to the Emmanuel Movement

n 1925, anticipating Worcester's retirement as Rector of the Emmanuel Church in 1929, Courtenay Baylor proposed to incorporate the traditions and methods of the Emmanuel Movement in the "Craigie Foundation." This would respect Worcester's wish not to exploit the name of the church after his retirement, and meetings would be held at 176 Marlborough Street, a few doors from Worcester's house. These premises were also the site where Baylor's alcohol groups were holding their meetings. Unfortunately, data about the Craigie Foundation are scanty after 1929, including an undated brochure, obtained from the Episcopal Diocesan Archives. This leaflet announces its program by stating its general aims: the Foundation would be "protected from the drawbacks of a popular movement"—meaning the risks of excessive publicity—and would therefore "not raise funds in any public way." Its purposes were:

> providing free of charge to whomsoever may apply for and be found to be in need of the following: individual psychotherapy . . . through psychological analysis and through the development of morale by means of psycho-therapeutic re-education and social therapy, that is, the correction of family or community maladjustments by means of . . . practical psychotherapy.

This redundant message recalled Worcester's early years, and even William James's emphasis on "practical fruits" rather than religion. There was no mention of alcoholism, which had become a specialty of Baylor's, nor of group-meetings as a specific method of treatment. Nevertheless Baylor continued to treat patients under the auspices of the "Craigie Foundation," at 176 Marlborough Street, at least until 1933, and probably longer. As far as we know, Baylor maintained the Emmanuel Movement's tradition of provid-ing free psychotherapy to the general public. During the depression he used funds from his private patients to main-tain the clinic, and he continued his private case-work from his offices in the Myles Standish Hotel at Kenmore Square, now one of nearby Boston University's dormitories. In 1944, two years before his death, he was invited to come back and resume his former volunteer position at the Emmanuel Church.

Courtenay Baylor (1870–1947), an important but now forgotten figure in the Emmanuel Movement, had been invaluable to Worcester, as a close collaborator over several decades. During those years he was apparently well-known for his special contributions to the treatment of alcoholism. Present-day interest in Baylor, for the history of alcohol-treatment, lies in his role as a lay leader in the group-therapy movement. He was the exemplary ex-patient who became a mentor and leader of the group by resolving his own alcohol problem successfully. And yet, as a public figure, he remains an elusive one for research, largely over-shadowed by his wife, a successful professional woman and a professor of social work at Simmons College. Besides Worcester's accounts of their work together, and a few newspaper clippings, we have only his 1919 book, *Remaking a Man*[1], and one article in a Simmons College social work journal.[2]

Baylor's book, subtitled "One Successful Method of Mental Refitting," began with a bold defense of his role as a layman, addressing the reader in non-technical language. He hoped to prove that "it is logical, legitimate, ethical and safe for one who has no medical or surgical knowledge and who has no psychological degrees to do a certain type of work in conjunction with skilled physicians." Having worked seven years with Worcester, he wrote, he had treated some thousand patients, with successful results in two-thirds. He had worked primarily with alcoholics, those suffering from what he called "an alcoholic neurosis," who wished to stop drinking but were unable to do so because of a "mental conflict." Gradually he had found that the same methods were effective with other neuroses, and es-pecially with returning soldiers from the First World War, "suffering from the neurotic conditions known as 'shell shock'." He also treated other members of the patients' family, attempting to "'cure'. . . an environment which has contributed to [the patient's] own abnormal nervous condi-tion." This approach can now be recognized as a pioneer form of "family psychotherapy."

Baylor's common-sense psychotherapy resembled Worcester's, with the same use of "direct and indirect sug-gestion, to calm racing thoughts." There was an appeal for free-associations ("what are you thinking about at this moment?") and childhood memories, in order to engage the patient's *unconscious* wish to change. There were also elements of Pratt's "relaxation exercises" and the term "re-education" was used. What stands out in Baylor's approach to the patient, however, is his strong emphasis on minimizing guilt, by disarming the alcoholic's expectation of being scolded or preached at, and the therapist's systematic avoidance of moralizing attitudes toward all patients. In this he was following Worcester's Biblical injunction, "resist not evil," in order not to evoke resistance to healing.

This element in both Baylor's and Worcester's psychotherapy, the rejection of guilt-provoking exhortations, was noted by Clinebell[3] and other writers on the history of alcoholism. Compared with moralistic approaches to alcoholism, like the Salvation Army, Clinebell called the Emmanuel Movement "the first pioneering attempt to treat alcoholism with a combination of individual and group psychotherapy." There are similarities in the methods of Alcoholics Anonymous, in the group-approach and in Baylor's use of himself, an ex-patient, as the group-leader, just as Ernest Jacoby had done before him. The tradition of the lay-leader also had traditional roots in religious sects like the Quakers, where each member of the congregation had acted as his own minister and there was no priestly hierarchy.

Despite the resemblance between Jacoby's and Baylor's group-meetings for alcoholics and Alcoholics Anonymous, there is no evidence for any direct connection. They overlapped in time, in that the first historic meeting of AA, according to "William W" [Wilson],[4] one of its founders, took place in 1935. This was on Mother's Day in Akron, Ohio, when he and "Doctor Bob" sat down at "W's" kitchen table. The antecedents of AA include references to a Dr. William Silkworth, a former alcoholic who had been cured by Carl Jung and became a specialist in the treatment of alcoholism. There had also been an encounter with a member of the Oxford Group, a Protestant revival movement that held meetings at the Calvary Episcopal Church in New York. During the heyday of the Emmanuel Movement, from 1908 to 1916, there had been Episcopal churches in New York and Brooklyn that established church clinics and group-meetings modeled on Worcester's methods. But there is no indication that any of these had any contact with the Oxford Movement. A church setting was also unlikely because an important feature of AA was the elimination of all explicit religious elements from the group-meetings.

One direct contribution of the Emmanuel Movement to alcohol treatment, however, and specifically of Baylor's work, was in the career of Richard Peabody.[5] Peabody had also been an ex-patient who became a lay-practitioner of alcohol treatment. He came from an eccentric and well-connected Boston family. His uncle was the Rev. Endicott Peabody, headmaster of Groton Academy. His first wife, Caresse, divorced him and married Harry Crosby, a nephew of J. P. Morgan; together they became *avant garde* publishers in the expatriate literary Paris of the 1920s.[6] Peabody sought treatment for his alcoholism at the Emmanuel Church in 1922, and according to McCarthy he was probably "Courtenay Baylor's most famous patient." Peabody was soon treating patients in Boston during the midtwenties, from an office on Newbury Street, not far from the Emmanuel Church, and he later moved to New York. He published articles in both magazines and medical journals, and one popular book, *The Commonsense of Drinking*.[7] In it Peabody paid homage to Baylor, but made no mention of the Emmanuel Movement. His book became better known than Baylor's book of ten years before, perhaps because the speakeasy era of the 1920s created a larger audience. Although Peabody had assimilated some theories about alcohol-treatment from the Emmanuel Movement, he differed in other ways from Baylor, among them in charging high fees for his services. He also suffered from several lapses in sobriety before his early death in 1936.

Peabody's followers had considerable influence on the growing public interest in alcoholism during the late '30s and '40s, exemplified by Strecker and Chambers'[8] popular book. Free clinics were established by the Yale Center of Alcohol Studies and McCarthy's[9] researches in the archives of Alcoholics Anonymous have since yielded an amazing discovery. In William "W"'s personal copy of Peabody's book, he had written in the margin that Peabody "was as far as is known the first authority to state, "once an alcoholic, always an alcoholic," and to prove it by returning to drinking and dying of alcoholism." This aphorism later became one of the basic tenets of Alcoholics Anonymous.

Some information about Courtenay Baylor as a person comes from Mrs. Emmeline Dunne,[10] who had been a social work student of Baylor's wife, Mrs. Edith Hedges Baylor. Dunne met Mrs. Baylor after graduating from Boston University School of Religious Education and Social Work in 1931. Mrs. Baylor was then head of the children's department at the Simmons College School of Social Work, and director of research at the Boston Children's Aid Society. She had written several books, *Reconstructing Behavior in Youth*,[11] in collaboration with Drs. Healy and Bronner of Judge Baker Guidance Center, and *The Rehabilitation of Children*.[12] In the early 1930s, Mrs. Dunne became a close friend of both the Baylors, a relationship that lasted until Mrs. Baylor's death in 1946. She recalled Courtenay Baylor as "carrying on some kind of self-styled psychiatric work with inebriates," in an office adjoining their apartment in the Myles Standish Hotel. She thought his work was somehow connected with the counseling service at the Emmanuel Church. She remembered both the Baylors with great affection and admiration: "the word 'Brahmin' comes to mind, because of a certain look and personality, but they were unpretentious, genuine, easy-to-know." She had no recollection of the Emmanuel Movement itself, of the Rev. Elwood Worcester, or of the name "Craigie Foundation." She believed Courtenay Baylor himself died two or three years after his wife's death.

Although Courtenay Baylor was not a Boston Brahmin, he came from a complex, aristocratic Virginia family that had proliferated all over the South.[13] His father, Charles Gano Baylor (1826–1906), had been a Confederate officer who belonged to the Georgia Peace Party and ran the blockade to interview President Lincoln.[14] Courtenay Baylor's father's first cousin, Mrs. Frances Courtenay Baylor (1848–1920), was an unusual woman, a feminist and perhaps the best known member of the family at that time. Growing up in San Antonio, New Orleans and England, in the family of a regular Army officer, Mrs. Baylor began to publish popular novels in 1885, many based on contrasts between races and nationalities. She began with a play, *Petruchio Tamed,* and she was working on a novel called *The Matrimonial Coolie* at the time of her death.[15]

Baylor's father had married Louisa Wadsworth of Washington D. C., the daughter of a high-ranking naval officer, and they settled in Marion, Massachusetts, where Courtnay was born in 1870. "Denied a college education by family reverses," he attended a boarding school in Connecticut and at eighteen he began as an office boy in a Boston manufacturing firm. Working his way up to an important position in the insurance business, Baylor's life exemplified the typical American self-made man of that era. He considered this excellent preparation for the understanding of his fellow men and the practice of lay psychotherapy, when he began his work with Dr. Worcester in 1912. He was always proud of his position as a non-professional, despite his excessively deferential attitude toward the medical profession, in which he was following Worcester's frustrating pattern.

To those who knew Baylor, he was a remarkable personality, recalled with great affection by Constance Worcester, according to McCarthy, who interviewed her in the early 1980s. An anonymous former patient, who had been treated by Peabody and other prominent therapists, remembers Baylor with unusual warmth.[16] In his seventies, Baylor was called "one of the most illuminating and persuasive personalities I have ever met," by Dwight Anderson,[17] another ex-alcoholic who became a lay-therapist. Anderson described one of Baylor's relaxation-exercises as a spell-binding, quasi-hypnotic experience, moved by his "soothing beautiful voice that lulled you . . . but gave you confidence." This episode took place in the presence of Anderson's wife on a summer-time verandah after sailing, but Baylor assured him he could accomplish the same effect "in an interview, driving a car or in the subway, anywhere at all."

In his years of retirement, Worcester himself continued to be active as a psychotherapist and rejoiced in his freedom from preparing his weekly sermon. Besides his autobiography, he wrote several scholarly books, one of them on the history of the Immaculate Conception. He also began a series of three-day visits to New York City, almost weekly during 1930–1931, to meet with Dr. Frederick Peterson and his wife, who had formed a kind of religious study-group. During these visits Worcester lectured at Grace Church in New York and Trinity in Brooklyn, both of which had adopted Emmanuel Movement programs some twenty years before. He also saw a full day of individual psychotherapy patients at both churches.

Peterson had been an eminent New York neurologist and psychiatrist long before the First World War. By coincidence, he had been a mentor of A. A. Brill, the first American to call himself a psychoanalyst. In 1908 Brill was a young psychiatrist at Manhattan State Hospital, and Peterson was the first to urge him to go abroad and study psychoanalysis. He told Brill, "Why don't you go to Zurich, to Bleuler and Jung; they are doing that Freud stuff over there. I think you would like it."[18] We have no indication of Peterson's religious interests at that time, but over twenty years later, Worcester wrote enthusiastically about his meetings with the Petersons as if they had created a kind of spiritual group-therapy.

Oddly enough, Worcester's memoirs made no mention of his regular collaboration with Dr. Flanders Dunbar, which took place during these same years when he was often in New York. At that time Dunbar was pursuing her interests both in faith healing and in psychosomatic medicine, as director of a Joint Committee on Religion and Medicine at Columbia University. Worcester also made no reference to Dunbar's other associate, the Rev. Anton T. Boisen, often called "the father of pastoral counseling." Boisen, who had collaborated with Dunbar for a time, had once been a patient of Worcester's, when Boisen had a parish in Worcester, Massachusetts. He was suffering from a severe mental disorder, probably a psychosis, and commuted into Boston for individual treatment with Worcester; the outcome was apparently a therapeutic success.

These complex interrelations among Worcester, Dunbar and Boisen were drawn to my attention by Robert Charles Powell in 1978, when we were interviewing Constance Worcester together. This was a time when Miss Worcester's sister, Dr. Blandina Worcester (Mrs. Carroll Brewster), happened to be visiting. Dr. Worcester was startled by a question of Powell's about Flanders Dunbar, who had been her classmate at Bryn Mawr, indicating a strong aversion to discussing her. She refused to answer any questions about Dunbar, including any explanation of her distaste. Powell's brilliant dissertation,[19] on Dunbar and her place in the history of psychosomatic medicine, demonstrated the links between Dunbar's theological background, the pastoral counseling movement and psychoanalysis, during the early years of psychosomatic research.

Worcester died quietly in 1940 while still at work on a book in collaboration with Dr. Walter Franklin Pierce, *The Psychic Phenomena of the Bible.* This reflected his lifelong belief in Spiritualism and so-called paranormal phenomena, which co-existed with his adherence to scientific psychology. He was survived by his two daughters and a son, each of whom, in his or her own way, continued their father's tradition of offering medical, psychological and spiritual counsel to the public.

9

The Worcester Family, 1940 to the Present

Besides the work of Courtenay Baylor and the "Craigie Foundation," which has proved to be so elusive and difficult to trace, the lives of Elwood Worcester's children and grandchildren continued to reflect his interests in their own individual and sometime original ways.

Dr. Blandina Worcester (1902–1984), his youngest daughter, studied medicine in the years when it was still an unusual career for women. She first attended Bryn Mawr, where "for two years I reveled in Greek and Philosophy," and then decided that she preferred working with people rather than books. She transferred to Radcliffe for her last two years, graduating with the class of 1923, and earned her M.D. at Johns Hopkins in 1927. During her third year, she practiced medicine single-handed in "Bloody Breathit County," Kentucky, relying on "common sense and sewing-scissors" when her chest of textbooks and surgical instruments failed to arrive. She interned at Wisconsin General

Hospital and at Johns Hopkins, and obtained a residency in pediatrics at Bellevue Hospital, New York. Her supervisor had written in a letter of recommendation "I would rather have Dr. Worcester on my service than Beatrice Lillie," a great wit of that time.[1]

For more than thirty years Dr. Blandina Worcester worked on the Children's Medical Service at Bellevue, and in the New York University Medical School, becoming Professor of Clinical Pediatrics. In 1954 she was made director of pediatrics at the New York Infirmary for Women and Children, a pioneer hospital in the medical education of women, founded by the Blackwell sisters. In 1935 she married Carroll H. Brewster, an eminent New York attorney who died in 1952. They had two sons, Carroll Worcester Brewster, and Dr. John Gurdon Brewster, who is the Episcopal chaplain at Cornell, the only descendant of Elwood Worcester to become a clergyman. In a one-page biography of Blandina Worcester, written by her older sister in 1983,[2] Constance took credit for having urged her sister to study medicine. Dr. Worcester and her husband moved to Ridgefield, Connecticut in 1937, where she died in 1984, at the age of eighty-two.

As Elwood Worcester's daughter Blandina continued his medical interests directly, by becoming a physician, his younger son, David, carried out his interests as an educator. David became a professor of English and, at an early age, President of Hamilton College. His career was prematurely cut short by a brain-tumor at the age of thirty-six. Blandina's son, Carroll Brewster, followed a similar career path, and became president of Hobart and William Smith Colleges. Even in his recent retirement, Carroll Brewster continues his educational work with a philanthropic foundation devoted to helping teenage children.

Elwood Worcester's eldest son, Gurdon Saltonstall Worcester, represented the tradition of lay-psychotherapy in an unusual form. Gurdon was a chemist by professional training and an inventor, making discoveries that were patented and utilized in the paint and dye industries. But he also became an Adlerian psychotherapist, who practiced in New York for many years. His special interest was in the treatment of alcoholism, and he was proud of his successful clinical results with unusual and difficult cases. He also practiced in Boston, and occasionally took care of his father's psychotherapy patients, during his father's vacations. His interest in alcoholism recalled the important part that the Emmanuel Movement had played in the early treatment of alcoholics by Ernest Jacoby and Courtenay Baylor in 1911–12. He may well have known Courtenay Baylor and Richard Peabody during the 1930s.

Worcester's oldest child, Constance Rulison Worcester (1896-1986), may have been closest to her father, and continued many of his interests, chiefly in creating a kind of residential psychotherapy. This took the form of transforming their family house into a residence for mental patients, in essence inventing her own version of what came to be called a "halfway house." She carried out this enterprise in the immense brownstone house at 186 Marlborough Street, in Boston's Back Bay, which had been the Rectory and her father's family home since the 1910s.

Constance was born in Bethlehem, Pennsylvania, "in the bishop's palace, as we used to call it," when her father was teaching philosophy at Lehigh University.[3] She remembered her maternal grandfather, Bishop Rulison, who came to live with them just before he died: his prickly beard and his telling her parents, "don't make her sit on my knee if she doesn't want to." She recalled their house on Locust Street in Philadelphia, the move to Boston when she was eight, and how they stayed in a small hotel on Boylston Street until the Rectory was ready. James Jackson Putnam was a neighbor, several blocks down Marlborough street, and she played with Putnam's daughters, one of whom, Frances, became her best friend. In her vivid recollections of the Putnam house, she was struck by its bare, uncarpeted floors and scanty furnishings, compared to their own oriental rugs, and the Putnam children's frugal Sunday suppers of bread and milk.

For some inexplicable reason, Constance and her younger brother Gurdon were kept from reading until they were over eight years old. "We couldn't tell one word from another, and I was eleven before I got into Miss Winsor's," a private day-school for upper-class girls. She had a wonderful teacher, Miss Flint, and Constance could still quote verbatim a poem she had written at the age of eleven. But she was held back because she failed algebra, year after year for eight years, before she was allowed to graduate from Miss Winsor's School. She was told by Miss Winsor that she was "not college material," but she easily passed her College Board exams for Bryn Mawr, after a year in France with her Aunt Connie, where she "had a wonderful time."

At Bryn Mawr she studied English and philosophy for two years, 1915–17, but she complained about "no guidance at home or at school." She disliked zoology dissections and she objected to the psychology taught by a famous German professor who condemned all religions. When the United States entered the First World War, she took nurses' training at Columbia and served as an Army nurse in local American camps until the Armistice in 1918. Before her military service, she had fought "a great battle" with her father over her wish to transfer from Bryn Mawr to Radcliffe, where she could live at home and take the subway to Harvard Square. He finally agreed to her admission to Radcliffe in 1917, which she entered in 1918 after discharge from the Army. She completed her studies there, graduating with the class of 1921 and receiving her A.B. in 1922.

She was very happy at Radcliffe, and developed a keen interest in philosophy and psychology, studying with the great Prof. William Hocking who, with Prof. George Sarton, had founded the progressive Shady Hill School. She had planned to continue a career in psychology, and had taken a few courses toward a master's degree, when she was overtaken by "a terrible tragedy." Her Aunt Connie committed suicide in New York, by jumping from a window in the Roosevelt Hotel, "and I had a nervous breakdown that ruined my life." She described this illness at various times over the years as "one of the three shocks in my life," the first at Miss Winsor's when her best friend, Frances Putnam, died in 1913. The third shock was her brother Gurdon's death in 1981, with whom she had earlier identified as one of the two neglected children who were not taught to read.

Constance Worcester described her breakdown after her aunt's death partly as a "seizure, like shell-shock," and partly as a chronic pain syndrome, diagnosed as "erythromelalgia," from which she suffered for fifty-two years. Some features of this chronic pain suggested the classic neurasthenias of the late nineteenth century, from which, she said, her mother had also suffered. These were the same nervous conditions that her father had treated so successfully among his parishioners and patients, but surprisingly, she recalled, her father showed little interest in her nervous breakdown. She described its onset as

a sudden attack, this terrible seizure, sitting at the lunchtable three weeks after Aunt Connie died. I couldn't feel, I couldn't think, I couldn't talk. It was like something taking possession of you, in one of the two parts of the brain; all the good part was gone and something very bad had taken its place . . . After the shock I was in bed for two years, up at the farm.

She consulted "the famous Dr. [Frederick] Peterson in New York," who, as we have seen, had been a friend of her father's. He diagnosed her condition as "shell-shock," like the nervous symptoms suffered by many soldiers that he had seen in the Great War. He told her about treating them with "a powerful drug that causes a repetition of the experience, from which you recover." But he explained that this medication was not suitable for her and that the pains in her legs might last a very long time. Returning to Boston, the doctors at the Peter Bent Brigham had nothing to offer in terms of treatment. Dr. Peterson's impression of a "neurotic, functional condition" was confirmed, as Miss Worcester recalled, and the diagnosis of "erythromelalgia" was also made, which she defined by translating its Greek components: "red and painful limbs."

Finally she found Dr. Theodore Badger (1899–1980), who remained her personal physician for many decades. In later life, he was a charming elderly internist who had been a pioneer in the study of tuberculosis. He was associated with the Channing Home (1857–1958), and with the famous Thorndike Research Laboratory at Boston City Hospital. He was also known as a family physician, devoted to his patients as a life-long friend and advisor, one of the last physicians who continued to make house-visits. He also served as medical consultant to Miss Worcester's many chronically sick tenants, with their complex mental and physical disabilities.

In the last decades of her life, Dr. Badger was succeeded by Dr. Arthur S. Pier, who remained her personal physician and consultant to her tenants until her death. Dr. Pier's father had been Miss Worcester's English composition teacher at Radcliffe, and he became her tenant in the last decades of his life, dying in his early nineties. Dr. Pier represented the same unselfish nineteenth century New England tradition of James Jackson, in which, like a minister, the physician assumed a patient's care for life. Dr. Pier was deeply impressed by the care Miss Worcester gave her tenants, including his father, and he vividly recalled some of the more colorful and difficult cases whom he was asked to treat in her house.

Returning to the 1920s and Miss Worcester's long convalescence from her "shock," she felt she could not continue her graduate studies in psychology and she was obliged to admit that she had no other real aim at the time. She undertook various volunteer jobs, such as caring for and teaching a disabled child. She did proofreading at the *Atlantic Monthly*, a few blocks down Marlborough Street from her house, and she worked briefly in a medical laboratory "where they tortured animals and said it was for the good of humanity." Then her father bought her "a simple farmhouse" in Kennebunkport, Maine, where she lived for a time and took care of her mother, who was suffering from neurasthenia, "while my father went off around the world on his big game hunting trips." Later she raised dogs as a commercial business, and worked as a private secretary in Boston until her parents' deaths in 1940.

Her father died during a visit to his daughter Constance at Kennebunkport, and her mother died within a few months, during a fierce blizzard. Although Miss Worcester inherited the family house on Marlborough Street, which had been a gift to her father by his parishioners upon his retirement, the house had been rented to a family that managed rooming-houses in the Back Bay. At the time of her parents' deaths, she went to live with her sister Blandina in Ridgefield, Connecticut. (Her Kennebunkport house later burned to the ground, in 1958, destroying all of her books, pictures, rugs, family photos and correspondence.) After a year or so Miss Worcester moved back to Boston, and lived at 45 River Street, taking possession of the Marlborough Street house only much later. In the interval the family that rented the house had drastically remodeled it, to create rooms for 47 people. As she remembers, there were "soldiers, sailors and airmen, active duty people coming and going" as they had been during the war years.

She finally regained the house in 1949, after a bitter legal struggle with her tenants, the Moriartys. Then she gradually reduced the accommodations in the house to ten or twelve small apartments, each with its own refrigerator and minimal cooking facilities, which she rented at nominal rates to the needy and mentally ill. Her first new tenant had been a retired clergymen, whom she had cared for until the end of his life. "My father being a clergyman, and my mother the daughter of a bishop, I was brought up along those lines. I thought that was the thing to do: being kind to the poor and the downtrodden."

After the death of the retired minister, she turned to patients who were being discharged from state mental hospitals and had no place to live. Many of these residents had neurological disabilities, as well as chronic psychoses, exhibiting strange deformities and bizarre behavior. She took care of these "patients" with great sensitivity, a successful combination of gentleness and tact with a firm sense of discipline. She was patient with their quirks and idiosyncrasies, and imperturbable in a crisis. Their tenancies lasted for many years, even decades, like a kind of extended family, but Miss Worcester kept her own life completely separate. She lived in a spacious apartment on the second floor, with two bays of windows the full width of the house. Her bed was on the left side, her desk, sofa and living-space on the right, and her kitchen in a large walk-in closet. She shared these quarters with her dachshund, Galahad, who became both deaf and blind. She had lived in the house for seventy-two years, and she died there in 1986, of acute kidney failure, probably due to a ruptured aneurysm in a renal artery.

In her last years, she had remained vigorous and active,

managing her large house and its many difficult tenants without any outside help. According to Dr. Arthur Pier,[5] her physician and friend, her mind was clear until her last illness; he called her "a saint who loved her 'patients' and saw to it that they were comfortable and well taken care of." She had suffered from increasing arthritis in her knees, and complications of cataract surgery had left her blind in one eye, but these physical afflictions did not diminish her energy, her lively conversation and her interest in what was going on in the world.

She had often talked about making provisions for the care of her sick tenants after her death, but she knew that the world had changed since she created her half-way house in 1949. She knew that the right person would be hard to find, who could—or would want to—manage a specialized rooming-house at the low rents she charged. She began to transfer some of her most disabled patients to nursing and retirement homes, whenever possible, beginning with those who had guardianships or trust-funds managed by a bank. One elderly Greek man, for example, developed a paranoid psychosis that required hospitalization, before he could finally be placed in a Greek old-age home. In short, she was also firm and decisive with her clients when necessary.

In replacing her sick patients with ordinary tenants, however, the modern world overtook her in many painful and disappointing ways. One of her most engaging new tenants, a young law-student, proved to be a thief and an impostor, who stole her silver and the family jewelry. Several other tenants were drug-dealers, and all her new tenants took advantage of her low rents. When she died rather suddenly, after a short hospitalization, the house was instantly taken over by its new tenants, who vandalized her apartment and destroyed her property. Even the few books and papers that Miss Worcester's two nephews had retrieved from the wreckage and put aside to be picked up, had vanished by the next morning. A coalition of these tenants resisted all efforts to evict them, and her nephews, Carroll and John Gurdon Brewster, heirs to her estate, were unable to take possession of the house. The legal costs and the tax penalties for pursuing eviction-proceedings were such that the Brewsters surrendered the house to a neighborhood association that agreed to keep it as a charitable foundation and maintain it as a rooming-house.

10

The Emmanuel Movement in Retrospect: Summary and Conclusions

T he Emmanuel Movement has been re-examined in its relation to other events in the first decade of this century: the popular psychotherapies of suggestion, the New England tradition of "medical psychotherapy," and the advent of psychoanalysis. Now let us consider what the significance of the Emmanuel Movement really was, besides its important role in the origins of group-therapy. Can this distant episode in the evolution of American "modernism" help us to understand certain characteristics of our native psychotherapy movements, and how they differed from corresponding events in Europe?

Free Psychotherapy and the "Class Method"

The special features of the Emmanuel Movement are easy to summarize, but its lasting influences are more difficult to assess. First, it was an early experiment in "community psychotherapy," in offering free treatment to one and all, regardless of social class or religious denomination. Under the unlikely auspices of a traditional Episcopal church in a fashionable neighborhood, the Rectory of the Emmanuel Church became virtually a psychiatric outpatient clinic for the treatment of the common neuroses. This occurred at a time when psychiatrists rarely had office practices, and most of them were engaged in the custodial care of chronic psychoses, in isolated mental hospitals, public and private. There was an increased demand for psychotherapy of everyday nervous conditions that was inadequately met by general physicians, neurologists, and a few psychologists who had a special interest in "abnormal psychology." Hospital out-patient clinics were struggling to provide medical treatment for Boston's rapidly increasing poor and immigrant population. The gap between supply and demand, for the treatment of both medical and nervous conditions, was being partially filled by many varieties of faith healing, like Christian Science, which was then at its peak of popularity.

The psychotherapy offered by the Emmanuel Movement was based on the new methods of suggestion, derived from Charcot and other French neurologists. Hypnosis, "waking suggestion" and "moral re-education" were used by Worcester and McComb, who were trained as clinical psychologists. Their individual methods of treatment were indistinguishable from the psychotherapy practiced by other psychologists like William James, by neurologists like James Jackson Putnam and Morton Prince, and by general physicians like William Edes.

Besides individual treatment, the chief innovation of the Emmanuel Movement was its use of weekly discussion-groups, a form of group-therapy that Worcester first applied to the treatment of neuroses in 1906. Worcester had adapted this approach, called the "class method," from his work with Dr. Joseph Pratt the year before, when they collaborated in creating a home-care program for tuberculosis patients who were too poor or too sick to be hospitalized. Pratt is rightly considered "the father of group psychotherapy" for his tuberculosis classes of 1905, but he himself never applied his "class method" to the treatment of nervous conditions until 1929, when he became chief of the medical clinic at the Boston Dispensary, then on Bennett Street. From Pratt's simple, quasi-authoritarian use of group-suggestion, "like a father surrounded by his children," as Worcester described him, the many varieties of group psychotherapy evolved from the 1930s up to the present. Many types of group-therapy seemed to emerge independently in different cities, like Trigant Burrow[1] in Baltimore, as if the United States were a fertile soil for the spontaneous generation of group experimentation.

Worcester's originality lay in applying Pratt's "class method" to the neuroses almost twenty-five years before Pratt did, and the "weekly group discussion" remained an essential element in the Emmanuel Movement's program until Worcester's retirement in 1929. The group meetings became even more important in the psychotherapy of Worcester's associate and successor, Courtenay Baylor, for at least another decade. But in Worcester's later writings in the early 1930s, there is no explicit emphasis on the unique contribution of the group meetings, in combination with individual treatment. Even in Baylor's 1919 book on alcoholism,[2] the group meetings were not specifically mentioned, as if they were taken for granted.

Nevertheless, despite the absence of fuller data, we may reasonably conclude that Worcester's most lasting contribution to the group therapy movement was made through the work of his lay followers, Jacoby and Baylor. Working with alcoholics as early as 1911, they had recognized the therapeutic value of relatively small peer groups, in which the leader was an ex-patient, as well as a non-professional, addressing his fellow-alcoholics as equals. This was in contrast to the regular weekly meetings of the Emmanuel

Movement, at which didactic and inspirational lectures were given by Worcester and his associates to relatively large groups, followed by group discussion, testimonials and a concluding hymn. Baylor also recognized quite early the importance of removing the weekly alcohol group from the church premises, thus emphasizing its secular nature. These essential elements, of a peer group led by a fellow patient, foreshadowed the group methods of Alcoholics Anonymous and other later self-help groups for drug-addicts. The first meeting of AA began in 1935, in Akron, Ohio, apparently unrelated to the Emmanuel Movement.

Religion and Medicine

Besides the use of groups, two other features distinguished the Emmanuel Movement from other psychotherapies of the time: Worcester's close working-relationship with physicians, and his use of clergymen and non-physicians in treating patients. Both features reflected strong, pre-existing convictions of Worcester's, but only a few physicians shared his views, and Worcester's use of lay-therapists evoked violent attacks from the medical Establishment. Worcester's post-graduate studies in Leipzig had trained him as a psychologist, and he had taught psychology for seven years at Lehigh University. But, when he came to Boston, he did not seek collaborators interested in psychotherapy among his fellow psychologists.

Instead he turned to physicians, in looking for a new project for his parish, and he found Dr. Joseph Pratt, who, by coincidence, was looking for a collaborator in his unorthodox methods of treating tuberculosis. Worcester had previously been influenced by Weir Mitchell in Philadelphia, and probably by his family medical traditions, going back to seventeenth century Puritan divines who had practiced both theology and medicine. These traditions may have influenced his determination to combine religion and medicine as reflected in the title of his first book. Worcester also found support for his medical interests in the history of early Christianity, when healing the sick was part of the bishop's traditional role.

But Worcester also believed that the spirit of the early Church could only be carried out by means of modern scientific methods. Scientific psychotherapy, at the turn of the century, meant the popular therapies of suggestion, with a pre-Freudian concept of the "subconscious mind," as practiced by Morton Prince and others and enthusiastically described in Prince's new *Journal of Abnormal Psychology*. Except for Worcester's assistant Dr. McComb, who was also a clergyman trained in clinical psychology, all of Worcester's early collaborators were in fact physicians. Pratt and Richard Cabot were young, ambitious internists with an idealistic zeal to help the impoverished immigrants who crowded Boston's out-patient clinics. Their interest in treating the common neuroses linked them with the New England tradition of "medical psychotherapy" and with older general physicians like Edes, George Gehring and Austen Riggs, all practicing their own variants of the psychotherapy of suggestion.

Worcester invited James Jackson Putnam to give the first lecture at the Emmanuel Church meetings, and Putnam remained sympathetic for several years, although he later withdrew from the Emmanuel Movement. He was an eminent neurologist, a leader in the psychotherapy movement and author of the first paper in English on Freud's "cathartic method." Through correspondence with Freud after the Clark Lectures in 1909, Putnam became Boston's first psychoanalyst. Isador Coriat was a close collaborator with Worcester and McComb and co-author of *Religion and Medicine*. He was an unusual psychiatrist whose career spanned the transition from the institutional care of the insane, under Adolf Meyer at Worcester State Hospital, to the psychotherapy of suggestion with Morton Prince. He eventually became Boston's second psychoanalyst, after Putnam's death in 1918.

The Assault on Lay Psychotherapy

Worcester's use of non-physicians as psychotherapists became the chief focus of attacks on the Emmanuel Movement by the medical Establishment, first in Boston and later in other cities. These attacks were virulent and unrelenting, and Worcester made strenuous efforts to meet medical objections. He hoped to disarm his critics by appointing a board of eminent physicians to ensure the correct differential diagnosis of organic and functional psychotherapy, and agreed to accept referrals only from physicians. But his emphasis on "medical control" failed to satisfy his enemies, and in 1910–1912 Worcester made a deliberate decision to withdraw from public notice. Nevertheless he continued his therapeutic work unobtrusively until his retirement in 1929.

Besides the effect of these attacks on the Emmanuel Movement, the battles over lay-psychotherapy may have a more general interest for the present-day reader. The typically American antipathy to treatment by non-physicians, with its many sources of conflict, its contradictions and odd bedfellows allied on opposite sides of these controversies, is interwoven with other cultural cross-currents at the turn of the century. Such unwavering antipathy to such a small number of psychotherapists implies, of course, an American public that was strongly attracted to non-medical forms of treatment. Nineteenth century American history, as Hofstadter[3] and others have shown, provides a showcase of unconventional therapies, from religious healing cults and Spiritualism to quasi-scientific diets, exercises, and massage. Europe had its religious shrines, its spas and traditions of "taking the waters," and created the phrenology and homeopathy movements, which were exported to our shores and flourished here too. But the American pursuit of successive health-fads seems to exhibit a special intensity, similar to our passion for a myriad of religious sects. Perhaps the recurrent waves of both secular and religious enthusiasms are all derived from our true religion: the American passion for self-improvement from the early Republic to the present. Even today the American appetite for "unconventional medicine" is substantial. Eisenberg, Kessler and their associates[4] recently reported that thirty-four percent of all medical patients make use of "alternative" forms of therapy. Most of these patients seek unorthodox cures while continuing to consult their traditional physicians, whom they rarely inform about their dabbling in chiropracty, "spiritual healing" and transcendental meditation.

In the Boston of the 1890s, medical authorities were preoccupied with quacks and untrained physicians, and the Massachusetts Medical Society supported legislation intended to prevent any non-physician from practicing psychotherapy. William James, then at the height of his popularity, was fiercely opposed to legal interference in the practice of faith-healing,[5] and he proclaimed that its clinical results deserved scientific study. In 1898, Putnam was one of the few prominent physicians to support James's position, although he admitted some ambivalence to James, his friend and former mentor.[6] Putnam wrote back that he opposed restrictive legislation that would interfere with James's research, but he admitted that he disliked all "mind curers" and was better able as a physician to see "their fanatical spirit . . . and the harm they sometimes do."

These legal efforts by the medical establishment to restrict lay therapy were prompted, in part, by the recent rise in popularity of the Christian Science Church, as well as other forms of non-medical healing like Horatio Dresser's New Thought movement. James, on the contrary, accepted all healers as members of the "mind-cure movement," from miracle-cures at religious shrines to the most scientific therapies of suggestion practiced by himself and his colleagues. The success of Christian Science was a significant social phenomenon, in satisfying a growing public need for psychotherapy of the common neuroses that the medical profession had largely failed to provide. A few leaders of the psychotherapy movement, like Edes and Putnam, had acknowledged this deficiency and urged more psychological teaching in medical education. Other physicians, like Richard Cabot,[7] were outspoken enemies of Christian Science, claiming that the church had set back the advent of scientific psychotherapy by many years.

Worcester clearly regarded the Emmanuel Movement as an effort to fulfill the public's increased need for treatment. Through its combination of religion and scientific medicine, he hoped to become an opposing force against the unscientific (and anti-medical) forms of faith-healing like Christian Science. The majority of physicians, however, refused to accept Worcester's fine distinctions and rejected the Emmanuel Movement because non-physicians were "still treating patients." Most physicians seemed unconcerned that the medical profession was unable to treat these patients, or that they were being treated free of charge. Putnam's vacillations over lay-psychotherapy reflected both his shy, fastidious, excessively modest traits and his personal transition between the psychotherapy movement and his conversion to psychoanalysis.

Between his address to the first Emmanuel "class" in 1906 and his withdrawal from the Movement in 1909, to join the "compact majority" of physicians opposed to lay-psychotherapy, Putnam followed a tortuous path. Its course was marked by newspaper statements, a lengthy essay in the *Harvard Theological Review*[8] and a painfully apologetic personal letter to Dr. Worcester.[9] Putnam had been one of the few physicians who acknowledged that Worcester and McComb were psychologists, as well as clergymen, but he still objected to their practicing psychotherapy. And Putnam saw no contradiction in accepting the right of James, Sidis, Münsterberg and other psychologists to practice psychotherapy, simply because the number of clinical psychologists was too small to become "a new medical specialty." Putnam thus came to disagree with James, his old teacher, who had admired and supported the Emmanuel Movement and deplored its destruction by excessive newspaper publicity. Putnam's own extreme distaste for publicity probably also contributed to his withdrawal from the Emmanuel Movement.

In 1909 another unexpected bedfellow joined the medical alliance against the Emmanuel Movement, when Sigmund Freud arrived in the United States to give his introductory lectures at Clark University. Because the Emmanuel Movement controversy was at its height, Freud was asked in his first newspaper interview what he thought of it. Unhesitatingly he rejected the Emmanuel Movement, aligning himself with his most conservative fellow physicians. This seemed ironic, in view of Freud's life-long defense of lay-analysis, his rejection of our American "medical fixation," and the fact that he had just welcomed the Rev. Pfister, a Swiss clergyman, as a fellow analyst. But this was a transitional period in Freud's career, when he was attempting to define the unique features of psychoanalysis. With the help of Ernest Jones, Freud showed that analysis was based on free association rather than hypnosis, and thus differed from all the other popular therapies of suggestion. But his American audience, on the contrary, was eager to welcome him and his therapy as just one more of many, perhaps improved, forms of hypnotic suggestion.[10]

This is not the place for a lengthy digression into the complex history of American psychoanalysis, with its decades-long conflicts over lay-analysis and their very recent resolution. But it would be fair to suggest that a few other elements probably entered into Freud's negative opinion about the Emmanuel Movement. One was his idiosyncratic aversion to all things American, especially its sensational press, and what Freud saw as the danger of popularizing and diluting the basic tenets of psychoanalysis. Another was his life-long rejection of religion in all its forms, which he expressed in his interview with the Boston *Evening Transcript* reporter.[11] Freud was dismissive of psychotherapy, and linked it with faith-healing as satisfying a basic human need for "mystery and authority," perhaps paraphrasing Dostoevski's famous scene with the Grand Inquisitor.

Freud's last comments on the Emmanuel Movement,[12] in reply to the Rev. Greene's inquiry, express the same world-weary distaste for both religion and American attitudes. He wrote that he deeply regretted that "so much energy in America has been poured forth in these religious movements." These words echo similar sentiments in Freud's contemporary letter to Arnold Zweig,[13] condemning Israel (then Palestine) as a land that has "never produced anything but religions, sacred frenzies, presumptuous attempts to overcome the outer world of appearance by means of the inner world of wishful thinking." In other words, Freud's anti-religious sentiments were not exclusively directed toward the United States.

In summing up features of the Emmanuel Movement that help to understand psychotherapy in the United States, compared to similar developments in Europe, we return to William James'[14] emphasis on the "practical fruits" of the mind-cure movement. His words apply to the Emmanuel Movement, as a prominent but short-lived example of the pre-analytic psychotherapy movement. James said that psychotherapy appealed to the "extremely practical turn of character of the American people," and represented "perhaps their only decidedly original contribution to the systematic philosophy of life . . . so intimately knit up with concrete therapeutics." Worcester, as a self-avowed "practical mystic," had learned from Pratt's "class method" of treating tuberculosis, and combined it with two pre-existing social phenomena: 1) the "modern" use of the church as a cultural and intellectual center, as well as a religious one, and 2) the local Boston passion for attending public lectures. What Burnham,[15] Hale[16] and others have said about American receptiveness to psychoanalysis applies equally to the Emmanuel Movement and other psychotherapies of suggestion, which were all welcomed as offering an optimistic, environmentalist view of mental illness as treatable, in contrast to gloomy nineteenth century German and Italian theories of "hereditary degeneration."

All these elements can be recognized in the writings of the time, the cheery moralism, the altruism and the worship of fresh air and outdoor living, as a series of quasi-religious observances. Even in their secularized form, the homiletic, "uplifting" style of Worcester, as well as Cabot and Pratt, suggest denatured derivatives of New England Calvinism. Putnam later struggled to convert Freud and Ernest Jones to a neo-Hegelian philosophy that would add an ethical dimension to psychoanalysis. His efforts were not successful but they represented, to Freud and Jones as self-avowed non-believers, another example of the lingering grip that religion had on American cultural life. In contrast, Freud and most European physicians, whatever their original religious backgrounds, were generally non-believers who adhered without conflict to their belief in science.

Following Pratt's 1905 tuberculosis class, the Emmanuel Movement made the first known use of group psychotherapy. This may indeed represent America's "only decidedly original contribution" to psychotherapy, despite the claims to priority of Moreno. But equally American, and even "modern," was the dramatic course of the Emmanuel Movement, its rapid rise in popularity, its short but intense period of flowering, and its abrupt decline, partly self-imposed, all within the brief period of 1906–1912. This drama of a rise and fall, as we know, was *caused* by the implacable enmity of the medical Establishment toward lay-psychotherapy. But its impact on the public was certainly *amplified* by the new journalism, already equipped with opinion-polls, feature articles on public controversies and interviews with visiting notables. Once the stage-lights of newspaper publicity had been turned off, by Worcester's deliberate self-effacement, the Emmanuel Movement quietly continued to perform useful services, on its own merits, for another three decades.

Freudian psychoanalysis superseded the Emmanuel Movement, as well as other variants of suggestive psychotherapy, by the 1920s. And eventually, almost fifty years later, the analytic community has finally laid to rest its ceaseless ancient struggle against lay analysis. From this vantage-point we can conclude that Freud and Putnam were probably short-sighted in rejecting the Emmanuel Movement, or at least in rejecting lay-psychotherapy. But as the analytic movement passes through its own periods of rapid, exuberant growth and its relative recent decline, Freud's original fear of American newspaper publicity comes back to life. Perhaps his fear of popularization, with its power to inflate and distort, may prove to be one of his apprehensions about the United States that was justified.

In looking back on the events of 1905–1912, on America's successive enthusiasms for the psychotherapies of suggestion, the Emmanuel Movement and psychoanalysis, we may see more elements in common than the differences that were once so fiercely disputed. Our forefathers' optimism often seems naïve in retrospect, as though looking back nostalgically on ancient revolutionary political movements. But there is an undeniable appeal in their very naïveté, in their belief in future progress, and a satisfaction in recalling men and women who lived through those events up to the present day.

Notes

Preface

1. George E. Gifford, Jr. ed., *Psychoanalysis, Psychotherapy and the New England Medical Scene 1894–1929* (New York: Science History Publications, 1978).

2. Russell G. Vasile, *James Jackson Putnam. From Neurology to Psychoanalysis* (Oceanside, NY: Dabor Science Publications, 1977).

3. Nathan G. Hale, Jr., *James Jackson Putnam and Psychoanalysis* (Cambridge: Harvard University Press, 1971); *Freud and the Americans. The Beginnings of Psychoanalysis in the United States 1876–1917* (New York: Oxford University Press, 1971).

Chapter 1

1. Nathan G. Hale, Jr., *Freud and the Americans.*

2. Estelle Shane, "Proposal on Non-Medical Training Approved," *Newsletter American Psychoanalytic Association* 19 (1988): 1, 10.

3. George M. Beard, *Sexual Neurasthenia*, 5th edition (New York: E. B. Treat, 1898). See also his *American Nervousness, Its Causes and Consequences* (New York: Putnam, 1881).

4. William James, "The Hidden Self," *Scribner's Magazine* 7 (1890): 361–373.

5. Sigmund Freud, *Five Lectures on Psychoanalysis,* in Sigmund Freud, *Works,* Standard Edition (London: Hogarth Press, 1957), vol. 11, 9–55.

6. Richard Hofstadter, *The Age of Reform* (New York: Random House, 1955).

Chapter 2

1. Elwood Worcester, *Life's Adventure* (New York: Scribner's, 1932).

2. Marguerite Beck Block, *The New Church in the New World. A Study of Swedenborgianism in America* (New York: Holt, Rinehart & Winston, 1932; reprinted, New York: Octagon Books, 1968).

3. *Dictionary of American Biography* (New York: Scribner's, 1928), vol. 20, 526–531.

4. Margaret Beck Block, *The New Church in the New World.*

5. David Freeman Worcester, "The Story of a Young American One Hundred Years Ago." Unpublished manuscript, 1932, typescript by Constance Worcester. A copy is in the author's possession, and another has been deposited in the Francis A. Countway Library of Medicine.

6. William James, *The Letters of William James, Edited by his Son Henry James* (Boston: Little, Brown & Co., 1926).

7. S. Weir Mitchell, *Doctor and Patient,* 3rd edition, (Philadelphia: J.B. Lippincott, 1896).

8. Stephan Thernstrom, *The Other Bostonians. Poverty and Progress in the American Metropolis, 1880–1970* (Cambridge: Harvard University Press, 1973).

9. Richard C. Cabot, *Social Service and the Art of Healing* (New York: Moffat, Yard and Co., 1909).

10. Roy Lubove, *The Professional Altruist. The Emergence of Social Work as a Career 1880- 1930* (Cambridge: Harvard University Press, 1965).

11. Katharine D. Hardwick, unpublished manuscript, quoted in Roy Lubove, *The Professional Altruist.*

12. William James, *The Varieties of Religious Experience* (New York: The Modern Library, 1929).

13. Pierre Janet, *The Major Symptoms of Hysteria* (London: Macmillan, 1906).

14. Josef Breuer and Sigmund Freud, *Studies in Hysteria,* In Sigmund Freud, *Works,* Standard Edition, vol. 2, 3–305.

15. Sigmund Freud, *Five Lectures on Psychoanalysis.*

16. Havelock Ellis, *Studies in the Psychology of Sex* (Philadelphia: F.A. Davis, 1901–1910), 6 v.

17. G. Stanley Hall, *Adolescence* (New York: D. Appleton, 1904).

18. Paul Dubois, *The Psychic Treatment of Nervous Disorders,* translated by Smith Ely Jelliffe and William A. White (New York: Funk & Wagnalls, 1906).

19. James Jackson Putnam, "Recent Experiences in the Study and Treatment of Hysteria at the Massachusetts General Hospital; with Remarks on Freud's Method of Treatment by 'Psycho-Analysis,'" *Journal of Abnormal Psychology* 1 (1909): 26–41.

20. Julius Silberger, *Mary Baker Eddy: An Interpretive Biography of the Founder of Christian Science* (Boston: Little, Brown, 1980).

21. William James correspondence: G. Stanley Hall to James, 27 December 1879 and James to Hall, 16 January 1880. Quoted in Ralph Barton Perry, *The Thought and Character of William James* (Boston: Little, Brown & Co., 1935), 2 volumes. Volume 2, pp. 18–19.

Chapter 3

1. Lawrence S. Kubie, *The Riggs Story: The Development of the Austen Riggs Center for the Study and Treatment of the Neuroses* (New York: Hoeber, 1960).

2. J. A. Curran, "Frederick Henry Gerrish, Maine's Outstanding Figure in Academic and Clinical Medicine, 1875–1920," *Journal of the Main Medical Association* 64 (1973): 47–50.

3. F. H. Gerrish, *Psychotherapeutics* (Boston: Badger, 1909).

4. Ernest Jones, *The Life and Works of Sigmund Freud* (New York: Basic Books, 1955), 2 v.

5. *Dictionary of American Biography,* vol. 7, 221–222.

6. Lawrence S. Kubie, *The Riggs Story*.

7. J. A. Curran, "Frederick Henry Gerrish, Maine's Outstanding Figure in Academic and Clinical Medicine, 1875–1920."

8. Joseph E. Garland, *An Experiment in Medicine* (Cambridge: Riverside Press, 1960).

9. Lawrence S. Kubie, *The Riggs Story*.

10. M. L. Cody, "Group Treatment of Psychoses by the Psychological Equivalent of the Revival," *Mental Hygiene* 15 (1931): 328–349.

11. Robert Herrick, *The Master of the Inn* (New York: Scribner's, 1908).

12. Max Eastman, *Enjoyment of Living* (New York: Harpers, 1948).

13. Robert T. Edes, "The New England Invalid," *Boston Medical and Surgical Journal* 133 (1895): 53–57, 77–81, 101–107.

14. Ibid.; see also Katherine Kish Sklar, *Catherine Beecher* (New Haven: Yale University Press, 1973).

15. James Jackson Putnam, "Not the Disease Only, But Also the Man," The Shattuck Lecture, 1899, *Medical Communications of the Massachusetts Medical Society* 18 (1899–1901), 58–9, 72.

16. *Dictionary of American Biography,* vol. 6, 18.

17. *Dictionary of American Biography,* vol. 2, 92–93.

18. George M. Beard, "The Longevity of Brain-Workers," *Quarterly Journal of Science,* n.s. 6 (1875): 430–449.

19. George M. Beard, *American Nervousness, Its Causes and Consequences*.

20. Boris Sidis, *The Psychology of Suggestion* (New York: Appleton, 1897).

21. Clarence P. Oberndorf, *A History of Psychoanalysis in America* (New York: Grune & Stratton, 1953).

22. Arthur J. Linenthal, *First a Dream: The History of Boston's Jewish Hospitals, 1896–1928* (Boston: Beth Israel Hospital and The Francis A. Countway Library of Medicine, 1990).

23. Eugene Taylor, "On the First Use of 'Psychoanalysis' at the Massachusetts General Hospital, 1903-05," *Journal of the History of Medicine and Allied Sciences* 42 (1988): 442–471.

24. James Jackson Putnam, "Recent Experiences in the Study and Treatment of Hysteria at the Massachusetts General Hospital."

25. Nathan G. Hale, Jr., *James Jackson Putnam and Psychoanalysis; Freud and the Americans.*

26. John C. Burnham, "Psychoanalysis and American Medicine, 1894–1910," *Psychological Issues Monograph 20* (New York: International Universities Press, 1967).

27. Eugene Taylor, "On the First Use of Psychoanalysis at the Massachusetts General Hospital, 1903–1905."

28. B. Sidis, M. Prince, and H. Linenthal, "A Contribution to the Pathology of Hysteria Based upon an Experimental Study of a Case of Hemianesthesia with Clonic Convulsive Attacks Simulating Jacksonian Epilepsy," *Boston Medical and Surgical Journal* 150 (1904): 674–678.

29. H. Linenthal and E. W. Taylor, "The Analytic Method in Psychotherapy," *Boston Medical and Surgical Journal* 155 (1906): 541–545.

30. Quoted in Arthur J. Linenthal, *First A Dream.*

31. Eugene Taylor, "The Controversial Beginnings of Hospital Social Service," *Focus, A Newsletter of the Harvard Medical Area* (April 18, 1983): 1–5.

32. *Dictionary of American Biography, Supplement Two* (New York: Scribner's, 1958), vol. 22, 83–85.

33. James Jackson Putnam to Elwood Worcester, September 12, 1908, Putnam Papers, The Francis A. Countway Library of Medicine.

34. Richard Cabot to James Jackson Putnam, September 21, 1908, Putnam Papers, The Francis A. Countway Library of Medicine.

35. Richard Cabot to James Jackson Putnam, February 17, 1911, Putnam Papers, The Francis A. Countway Library of Medicine.

Chapter 4

1. S. R. Slavson, "Pioneers in Group Psychotherapy: Joseph Hersey Pratt, M.D.," *International Journal of Psychotherapy* 1 (1951): 95–99.

2. J. H. Pratt, "The Class Method in the Home Treatment of

Pulmonary Tuberculosis," *Transactions of the American Climatological Association* 27 (1911): 87–118.

3. M. Rosenbaum, "Group Psychotherapy: A Historical Review," in B. B. Wolman, ed., *International Encyclopedia of Neurology, Psychiatry and Psychoanalysis* (New York: Van Nostrand-Reinhold, 1977).

4. S. B. Hadden, "Historic Background of Group Psychotherapy," *International Journal of Group Psychotherapy* 5 (1955): 162–168.

5. M. L. Cody, "Group Treatment of the Psychoses by the Psychological Equivalent of the Revival."

6. Trigant Burrow, "The Group Method of Analysis," *Psychoanalytic Review* 14 (1927): 268- 280.

7. E. W. Lazell, "Group Treatment of Dementia Praecox," *Psychoanalytic Review* 8 (1931): 168–179.

8. J. L. Moreno, "History of Group Psychotherapy," unpublished manuscript, 1960, Moreno Papers, The Francis A. Countway Library of Medicine.

9. J. H. Pratt, "An Attempt to Treat Consumption by Sanitarium Methods in the Homes of the Poor," *Journal of the Outdoor Life* (September 1905).

10. J. H. Pratt, "The Class Method of Treating Consumption in the Homes of the Poor," *Journal of the American Medical Association* 49 (1907): 755–759; "Results Obtained in the Treatment of Pulmonary Tuberculosis by the Class Method," *British Medical Journal* 2 (1908): 1070- 1071; "The Class Method in the Home Treatment of Pulmonary Tuberculosis."

11. May Sarton, *I Knew a Phoenix* (New York: Norton, 1979).

12. J. H. Pratt, "The Class Method of Treating Consumption in the Homes of the Poor."

13. J. H. Pratt, "The Principles of Class Treatment and Their Application to Various Chronic Diseases," *Hospital Social Service Review* 6 (1922): 401–411.

14. J. H. Pratt, "The Group Method in the Treatment of Psychomatic Disorders," *Psychodrama Monographs* 19 (1946); "The Use of Déjérine's Methods in the Treatment of the Common Neuroses by Group Psychotherapy," *Bulletin of the New England Medical Center* 15 (1953): 9–17.

15. J. Déjérine and E. Gaukler, *The Psychoneuroses and their Treatment by Psychotherapy*, translated by Smith Ely Jelliffe, (Philadelphia: J. B. Lippincott, 1913).

16. J. H. Pratt, "The Use of Déjérine's Methods in the Treatment of the Common Neuroses by Group Psychotherapy."

17. James Jackson, *Letters to a Young Physician Just Entering Upon Practice* (Boston: Phillips, Sampson & Co., 1855).

18. J. H. Pratt, "The Influence of the Emotions in the Causation and Cure of Psychoneuroses," *International Clinics* (1934).

19. Joseph H. Kaplan, Paul E. Johnson and Haldean Lindsey, Eds., *Fifty Years in Group Psychotheraphy: Commemorating the Pioneering of Joseph Hersey Pratt, M.D. 1905–1955* (Boston: New England Medical Center, 1955).

20. Richard Cabot, "Joseph H. Pratt, An Appreciation," In *Anniversary Volume on His Sixty-Fifth Birthday* (Lancaster, Pa, 1937).

21. Elwood Worcester, *Life's Adventure.*

22. G. W. Thomas, "Group Psychotherapy. A Review of Recent Literature," *Psychosomatic Medicine* 5 (1943): 166–180.

23. Herbert I. Harris, "Efficient Psychotherapy for the Large Outpatient Clinic," *New England Journal of Medicine* 221 (1939): 1–5.

24. S. R. Slavson, "Pioneer in Group Psychotherapy: Joseph Hersey Pratt, M.D."

25. J. H. Pratt to George Cheever Shattuck, 10 July 1945, The Francis A. Countway Library of Medicine

Chapter 5

1. Elwood Worcester, *Life's Adventure.*

2. Ibid.

3. Elwood Worcester, Samuel McComb and Isador H. Coriat, *Religion and Medicine. The Moral Control of Nervous Disorders* (New York: Moffat, Yard, 1908).

4. Elwood Worcester, *Religion and Medicine Publications* (New York: Moffat and Yard, 1908), nos. 1–9.

5. Elwood Worcester, *Life's Adventure.*

6. Ibid.

7. Elwood Worcester, Scrapbooks of clippings from the popular press on the Emmanuel Movement, 5 volumes (1906–1916), The Francis A. Countway Library of Medicine.

8. Barbara Sicherman, "Isador H. Coriat, The Making of an American Psychoanalyst," in George E. Gifford, Jr., ed., *Psychoanalysis, Psychotherapy and the New England Medical Scene, 1894–1944.*

9. Elwood Worcester, Samuel McComb and Isador H. Coriat, *Religion and Medicine.*

10. Ibid.

11. Isador H. Coriat, *Abnormal Psychology* (New York: Moffat, Yard, 1914).

12. Paul Dubois, *The Psychic Treatment of Nervous Disorders.*

13. Isador Coriat, *Abnormal Psychology.*

14. Boris Sidis, *The Psychology of Suggestion.*

15. Joseph Jastrow, *The Subconscious* (Boston: Houghton Mifflin Co., 1905).

16. Hugo Münsterberg, *Psychotherapy* (New York: Moffat, Yard, 1909).

17. Richard Hofstadter, *The Age of Reform.*

18. Robert Darnton, *Mesmerism and the End of the Englightenment in France* (Cambridge: Harvard University Press, 1968).

19. Richard Hofstadter, *The Age of Reform.*

20. Elwood Worcester, *Religion and Medicine Publications.*

21. William James, *The Energies of Men* (New York: Moffat, Yard, 1908).

22. Elwood Worcester, *Religion and Medicine Publications.*

Chapter 6

1. Elwood Worcester, Scrapbooks of clippings from the popular press on the Emmanuel Movement (1906–1916), 5 volumes.

2. Isador H. Coriat, Scrapbooks (1906–1953) 3 volumes. Clippings from United States and Canadian newspapers, magazines and medical journals. Boston Psychoanalytic Institute and The Francis A. Countway Library of Medicine.

3. Richard Cabot, "New Phases in the Relation of the Church to Health," *The Outlook* 88 (29 February 1908): 504–507.

4. Elwood Worcester, Scrapbooks of clippings from the popular press on the Emmanuel Movement, volume containing clippings of March, 1908.

5. W. B. Parker, ed., *Psychotherapy, A Course of Reading in Sound Psychology, Sound Medicine and Sound Religion* (New York: Center Publishing Co., 1908–1909).

6. Unsigned editorial, entitled "The Emmanuel Movement in Mental Healing", *Boston Medical and Surgical Journal* 159 (November, 26, 1908).

7. James Jackson Putnam, letters to the editor, *Boston Herald,* November 20, 1908.

8. James Jackson Putnam to Elwood Worcester, September, 12, 1908, Putnam Papers, The Francis A. Countway Library of Medicine.

9. James Jackson Putnam, "The Service to Nervous Invalids of the Physician and Minister," *Harvard Theological Review* 2 (1909): 235–250.

10. See unsigned editorial, "The Emmanuel Movement," *Medical Record*, November 31, 1908.

11. *Boston Globe,* December 27, 1908.

12. E. E. Southard, *Boston Globe,* December 27, 1908.

13. G. Stanley Hall, *Boston Herald,* December 30, 1908.

14. *Boston Globe,* January 29, 1909.

15. *Boston Medical and Surgical Journal,* February 16, 1909.

16. James Jackson Putnam, "The Service to Nervous Invalids of the Physician and Minister."

17. Nathan G. Hale, Jr., *James Jackson Putnam and Psychoanalysis;* also, *Freud and the Americans.*

18. James Jackson Putnam, *Human Motives* (Boston: Little, Brown, 1915).

19. Nathan G. Hale, Jr., *James Jackson Putnam and Psychoanalysis.*

20. James Jackson Putnam to Henry P. Walcott, January 10, 1910, Putnam Papers, The Francis A. Countway Library of Medicine.

21. John C. Burnham, *Psychoanalysis and American Medicine, 1894–1918.*

22. Sigmund Freud, "The Question of Lay Analysis," in Sigmund Freud, *Works,* Standard Edition (London: Hogarth Press, 1959), volume 20, 183–258.

23. Adelbert Albrecht, "Interview with Sigmund Freud," *Boston Evening Transcript,* September 11, 1909.

24. Richard Löwenfeld. This is an error by the journalist, Albrecht, because there is no trace of this name in the medical literature. Freud was probably referring to Leopold Löwenfeld, who had written many books about neurasthenia between 1894 and 1909. The book Freud referred to may well have been *Sexuelleben and Nervenleider: Die Nervöse Störungen Sexuellen Ursprungs* (Wiesbaden: J. F. Bergmann, 1899).

25. Sigmund Freud, *Minutes of the Vienna Psychoanalytic Society,* (New York: International Universities Press, 1967). Vol. 2 (1908–1910), entry for February 10, 1909.

26. John G. Greene, "The Emmanuel Movement 1906–1929," *New England Quarterly* 1 (1934): 494–532.

27. Sigmund Freud to J. G. Greene, 1934, translated by Ingrid B. Gifford, The Francis A. Countway Library of Medicine. Freud's letter was published in part in Ernest Jones' biography of Freud.

28. Sigmund Freud, *Letters of Sigmund Freud and Arnold Zweig,* Ernest Freud, ed. (New York: Harcourt Brace, 1970).

Chapter 7

1. Unsigned book review, *Lancet* 1 (February 13, 1909): 469–470.

2. John G. Greene, "The Emmanuel Movement, 1906–1929."

3. Lightner Witmer, "Review of *Religion and Medicine,*" *The Psychological Clinic* 2 (1908- 1909): 212–223, 239–249, 282–299.

4. M. Rosenbaum, "Group Psychotherapy: an Historical Review."

5. J. H. Pratt, quoted in "Tuberculosis Prevention," *New York Evening Post,* May 12, 1916.

6. John G. Greene, "The Emmanuel Movement, 1906–1929."

7. William James, *A Pluralistic Universe: Hibbert Lectures on the*

Present Situation in Philosophy (New York: Longmans, Green & Co., 1909).

8. William James to T. S. Perry, January 29, 1909. *The Letters of William James.*

9. William James to T. Flournoy, September 28, 1909. *The Letters of William James.*

10. Saul Rosenzweig, *The Historic Expedition to America* (St. Louis: Rana House, 1994), 171- 197. Dr. Rosenzweig provides a fresh and original interpretation of the historic encounter between Freud and William James at the Clark Lectures.

11. Elwood Worcester and Samuel McComb, *The Christian Religion as a Healing Power* (New York: Moffat, Yard, 1908).

12. Isador H. Coriat, *Abnormal Psychology.*

13. *New York Churchman,* Correspondent Column (unsigned), January 21, 1911.

14. *Boston Evening Transcript,* "Year's Work at Emmanuel," February 1, 1911.

15. John G. Greene, "The Emmanuel Movement, 1906–1929."

16. Edith A. Talbot, "The Rambler," column in *Boston Herald,* May 17, 1916.

Chapter 8

1. Courtenay Baylor, *Remaking a Man: One Successful Method of Mental Refitting* (New York: Moffat, Yard, 1919).

2. Courtenay Baylor, "An Approach to Work with the Individual," *The Social Worker* 8 (1931): 7–9.

3. H. J. Clinebell, Jr., *Understanding and Counseling the Alcoholic* (New York: Abingdon Press, 1956).

4. William "W" [Wilson], "The Society of Alcoholics Anonymous," *American Journal of Psychiatry* 106 (1949): 370–375.

5. Katherine McCarthy, "Psychotherapy and Religion: The Emmanuel Movement," *Journal of Religion and Health* 23 (1984): 92–105; "Early Alcoholism Treatment: The Emmanuel Movement and Richard Peabody," *Journal of Studies on Alcohol* 45 (1984): 59–73.

6. Caresse Crosby, *The Passionate Years, a Memoir* (New York: Dial Press, 1953). See also Geoffrey Wolff, *Black Sun. The Brief Transit*

and Violent Eclipse of Harry Crosby (New York: Random House, 1976). The Crosby's publishing house was The Black Sun Press.

7. Richard R. Peabody, *The Commonsense of Drinking* (Boston: Little, Brown, 1931).

8. E. A. Strecker and F. T. Chambers, Jr., *Alcohol: One Man's Meat* (New York: Macmillan, 1938).

9. Katherine McCarthy, "Psychotherapy and Religion: The Emmanuel Movement"; "Early Alcoholism Treatment: The Emmanuel Movement and Richard Peabody."

10. Emmeline Dunne, personal communications, 1978–1979.

11. William Healy, A. F. Bronner, E. M. H. Baylor and J. P. Murphy, *Reconstructing Behavior in Youth* (New York: Knopf, 1931).

12. E. M. H. Baylor and E. D. Marchesi, *The Rehabilitation of Children* (New York: Harpers, 1939).

13. Orval Walker Baylor, *Baylor's History of the Baylors* (Washington, D.C.: Leroy Printing Co., 1914).

14. Obituary in the *Boston Globe,* May 6, 1947.

15. *Dictionary of American Biography,* vol. 2, 76.

16. Katherine McCarthy, "Psychotherapy and Religion: The Emmanuel Movement"; "Early Alcoholism Treatment: The Emmanuel Movement and Richard Peabody."

17. Dwight Anderson, "The Place of the Lay Therapist in the Treatment of Alcoholics," *Quarterly Journal of Studies on Alcohol* 5 (1944): 257–266.

18. Nathan G. Hale, Jr., *Freud and the Americans.*

19. Robert Charles Powell, "Healing and Wholeness: Helen Flanders Dunbar (1909–1959) and an Extra-Medical Origin of the American Psychosomatic Movement (1906–1936)," Ph.D. dissertation, Department of History, Duke University, 1974.

Chapter 9

1. Blandina Worcester, audiotaped interview, 1984, plus subsequent correspondence. Radcliffe Alumnae Archives, Schlesinger Library, Harvard University

2. Radcliffe Alumnae Archives

3. Constance R. Worcester, personal communications, audiotaped interviews and one videotape, 1972–1985. Archives of the Boston Psychoanalytic Society/Institute.

4. Arthur S. Pier, personal communications to the author, 1992–1993.

Chapter 10

1. Trigant Burrow, "The Group Method of Psychoanalysis."

2. Courtenay Baylor, *Remaking a Man.*

3. Richard Hofstadter, *The Age of Reform.*

4. D. M. Eisenberg, R. C. Kessler, C. Foster, F. E. Norlock, D. R. Talkins and T. Delbanco, "Unconventional Medicine in the U.S. Prevalence, Costs & Patterns of Use," *The New England Journal of Medicine* 328 (1993): 246–252.

5. William James, *The Letters of William James.*

6. Nathan G. Hale, Jr., *James Jackson Putnam and Psychoanalysis.*

7. W. B. Parker, ed., *Psychotherapy, a Course of Reading in Sound Psychology, Sound Medicine and Sound Religion.*

8. James Jackson Putnam, "The Service to Nervous Invalids of the Physician and the Minister."

9. James Jackson Putnam to Elwood Worcester, September 12, 1908. Putnam Papers, The Francis A. Countway Library of Medicine.

10. Sanford Gifford, "The American Reception of Psychoanalysis, 1908–1922," in Adele Heller and Lois Rudnick, eds., *1915, The Cultural Moment* (New Brunswick, N.J.: Rutger's University Press, 1991), 128–145.

11. Adelbert Albrecht, "Interview with Sigmund Freud."

12. Sigmund Freud to J. G. Greene, 1934.

13. Sigmund Freud to Arnold Zweig in Ernest Freud, ed., *Letters of Sigmund Freud and Arnold Zweig.*

14. William James, *The Varieties of Religious Experience.*

15. John C. Burnham, "Psychoanalysis and American Medicine, 1894–1915."

16. Nathan G. Hale, Jr., *Freud and the Americans.*

145

Index

Index

Worcester, Rev. Elwood (*cont.*)
72, 74–76, 79–80, 82, 83, 84, 95,
96, 97, 105, 120–124, 126, 130;
Ordination and early church
work, 19–21; Relationship with
Richard C. Cabot, 44, 45–46, 65;
Relationship with Isador H. Coriat, 65, 76; Relationship with
Samuel McComb, 61–65, 74, 76;
Relationship with Joseph H.
Pratt, 50, 57, 59–60, 64, 65; Rela-
tionship with James J. Putnam,
79–80; Retirement, 99, 106–108;
University education, 16–19;
Use of lay therapists, 6; Views
on psychoanalysis, 97–98; *Body,
Mind and Spirit,* 96; *The Chris-
tian Religion as a Healing Power,*
94; *Life's Adventure,* 96; *The Psy-
chic Phenomena in the Bible,* 108;
Religion and Medicine, 65, 73, 79–
80, 89, 91, 96, 123
Worcester, Gurdon Saltonstall,
110–112
Worcester, Mary, 15
Worcester, Rev. Noah, 10
Worcester, Samuel Austin, 10–11
Worcester, Thomas, 10
Worcester State Hospital, 65, 123
Wundt, Wilhelm, 1, 16–17, 19, 90

Yale Center for Alcohol Studies,
104

Zweig, Arnold, 87, 128

About the Author

Sanford Gifford was born in Omaha, Nebraska, and grew up in Chicago. He attended Harvard College, Northwestern Medical School and interned at the University of California Hospital in San Francisco. After military service in the South Pacific, he took a Veterans Administration residency in Boston and completed his analytic training at the Boston Psychoanalytic Society/Institute. He was a psychiatrist at the Peter Bent Brigham Hospital from 1948 to 1993, when he resigned because of conflicts with managed care. He continues to work part time at the West Roxbury VA Hospital. He is Associate Clinical Professor of Psychiatry at Harvard Medical School, Director of the Library at the Boston Psychoanalytic Society/Institute, and Chairman of the History and Archives Committee of the American Psychoanalytic Association.